HLA and Disease

Editors

JULIO C. DELGADO
ESZTER LÁZÁR-MOLNÁR

CLINICS IN LABORATORY MEDICINE

www.labmed.theclinics.com

Editor-in-Chief
MILENKO JOVAN TANASIJEVIC

December 2018 • Volume 38 • Number 4

ELSEVIER

1600 John F. Kennedy Boulevard • Suite 1800 • Philadelphia, Pennsylvania, 19103-2899

http://www.theclinics.com

CLINICS IN LABORATORY MEDICINE Volume 38, Number 4
December 2018 ISSN 0272-2712, ISBN-13: 978-0-323-64220-0

Editor: Stacy Eastman
Developmental Editor: Laura Fisher

Reprints. For copies of 100 or more, of articles in this publication, please contact the Commercial Reprints Department, Elsevier Inc., 360 Park Avenue South, New York, New York 10010-1710. Tel. 212-633-3874, Fax: 212-633-3820, E-mail: reprints@elsevier.com.

Clinics in Laboratory Medicine (ISSN 0272-2712) is published quarterly by Elsevier Inc., 360 Park Avenue South, New York, NY 10010-1710. Months of issue are March, June, September, and December. Business and Editorial offices: 1600 John F. Kennedy Blvd., Suite 1800, Philadelphia, PA 19103-2899. Periodicals postage paid at NewYork, NY and additional mailing offices. Subscription prices are $263.00 per year (US individuals), $507.00 per year (US institutions), $100.00 per year (US students), $347.00 per year (Canadian individuals), $617.00 per year (Canadian institutions), $185.00 per year (Canadian students), $402.00 per year (international individuals), $617.00 per year (international institutions), $185.00 (international students). Foreign air speed delivery is included in all Clinics subscription prices. All prices are subject to change without notice. POSTMASTER: Send address changes to *Clinics in Laboratory Medicine*, Elsevier Health Sciences Division, Subscription Customer Service, 3251 Riverport Lane, Maryland Heights, MO 63043. **Customer Service: 1-800-654-2452 (US). From outside of the US and Canada, call 1-314-447-8871. Fax: 1-314-447-8029. E-mail: journalscustomerservice-usa@elsevier.com (for print support) or journalsonlinesupport-usa@elsevier.com (for online support).**

Clinics in Laboratory Medicine is covered in *EMBASE/Exerpta Medica, MEDLINE/PubMed (Index Medicus), Cinahl, Current Contents/Clinical Medicine, BIOSIS and ISI/BIOMED.*

Contributors

EDITOR-IN-CHIEF

MILENKO JOVAN TANASIJEVIC, MD, MBA
Vice Chair for Clinical Pathology and Quality, Department of Pathology, Director of Clinical Laboratories, Brigham and Women's Hospital, Dana-Farber Cancer Institute, Associate Professor of Pathology, Harvard Medical School, Boston, Massachusetts, USA

EDITORS

JULIO C. DELGADO, MD, MS
Professor of Pathology, University of Utah, Division Chief of Clinical Pathology, Chief Medical Officer, ARUP Laboratories, Salt Lake City, Utah

ESZTER LÁZÁR-MOLNÁR, PhD
Assistant Professor of Pathology, University of Utah, Director, Histocompatibility & Immunogenetics Laboratory, Medical Director, Immunology, ARUP Laboratories, Salt Lake City, Utah

AUTHORS

MEAGAN BARNER, CHS
Laboratory Supervisor, Kashi Clinical Laboratories, Portland, Oregon, USA

NILESH CHITNIS, PhD
Immunogenetics Fellow, Department of Pathology and Laboratory Medicine, The Children's Hospital of Philadelphia, Abramson Research Center, Philadelphia, Pennsylvania, USA

MATTHEW F. CUSICK, PhD, D(ABHI)
Assistant Professor, Director, Immune Evaluation Laboratory, Baylor College of Medicine, Houston, Texas, USA

JENEFER DEKONING, PhD
Scientific Director, Kashi Clinical Laboratories, Portland, Oregon, USA

MANISH J. GANDHI, MD
Associate Professor of Laboratory Medicine and Pathology, Division of Transfusion Medicine, Mayo Clinic, Rochester, Minnesota, USA

PHILLIP HALLORAN, MD, PhD
Director, Division of Nephrology and Transplant Immunology, Department of Medicine, University of Alberta, Founder, Alberta Transplant Applied Genomics Center, CEO, Transcriptome Sciences Inc, Edmonton, Alberta, Canada

ANDRÉS JARAMILLO, PhD
Director, Histocompatibility Laboratory, Associate Professor, Department of Laboratory Medicine and Pathology, Mayo Clinic, Phoenix, Arizona, USA

PETER T. JINDRA, PhD, D(ABHI)
Assistant Professor, Department of Surgery, Director, Immune Evaluation Laboratory, Baylor College of Medicine, Houston, Texas, USA

ZAHRA KASHI, PhD
Lab Director, CEO, Kashi Clinical Laboratories, Portland, Oregon, USA

ATTILA KUMÁNOVICS, MD
ARUP Institute for Clinical and Experimental Pathology, Department of Pathology, University of Utah School of Medicine, Salt Lake City, Utah, USA

ESZTER LÁZÁR-MOLNÁR, PhD
Assistant Professor, Department of Pathology, University of Utah School of Medicine, Salt Lake City, Utah, USA

DANMENG LI, MD
Laboratory Technician, Department of Pathology, Immunology and Laboratory Medicine, University of Florida College of Medicine, University of Florida, Gainesville, Florida, USA

DIMITRI MONOS, PhD
Professor, Department of Pathology and Laboratory Medicine, The Children's Hospital of Philadelphia, Perelman School of Medicine, University of Pennsylvania, Abramson Research Center, Philadelphia, Pennsylvania, USA

DAVID A. OSTROV, PhD
Associate Professor, Department of Pathology, Immunology and Laboratory Medicine, University of Florida College of Medicine, University of Florida, Gainesville, Florida, USA

TRACIE PROFAIZER, MS
ARUP Institute for Clinical and Experimental Pathology, Department of Pathology, University of Utah School of Medicine, Salt Lake City, Utah, USA

RAJA RAJALINGAM, PhD
Professor of Surgery, Director of Immunogenetics and Transplantation Laboratory, University of California, San Francisco, San Francisco, California, USA

DANIEL S. RAMON, PhD
Associate Director, Histocompatibility Laboratory, Assistant Professor, Department of Laboratory Medicine and Pathology, Mayo Clinic, Phoenix, Arizona, USA

CARRIE A. SCHINSTOCK, MD
Assistant Professor of Medicine, William J. von Liebig Center for Transplantation and Clinical Regeneration, Mayo Clinic, Rochester, Minnesota, USA

RYAN J. SCHUTTE, PhD
Postdoctoral Associate, Department of Pathology, Immunology and Laboratory Medicine, University of Florida College of Medicine, University of Florida, Gainesville, Florida, USA

MENGKAI SHIEH, MD
Visiting Scientist, Department of Pathology and Laboratory Medicine, The Children's Hospital of Philadelphia, Abramson Research Center, Philadelphia, Pennsylvania, USA

MELISSA SNYDER, PhD
Assistant Professor, Department of Laboratory Medicine and Pathology, Mayo Clinic, Rochester, Minnesota, USA

SCOTT T. STOLL, BS
Supervisor, Histocompatibility Laboratory, Department of Laboratory Medicine and Pathology, Mayo Clinic, Phoenix, Arizona, USA

YONGHU SUN, MD, PhD
Associate Professor, Department of Dermatology, Shandong Provincial Institute of Dermatology and Venereology, Jinan, Shandong, PR China

FUREN ZHANG, MD, PhD
Professor, Department of Dermatology, Shandong Provincial Institute of Dermatology and Venereology, Jinan, Shandong, PR China

Contents

Human leukocyte antigen (HLA) allele ambiguities are the result of limitations of current HLA typing methodologies. Ambiguities maybe due to polymorphisms in unsequenced regions of HLA genes or cis/trans variants that cannot be distinguished by Sanger sequencing. Next generation sequencing (NGS) can resolve these two sources of ambiguity because the entire gene can be sequenced. Commercially available HLA NGS genotyping kits enable laboratories to deliver high-quality and unambiguous HLA typing results at an affordable cost. Third generation sequencing technologies are poised to further improve sequencing quality, shorten turn-around and library preparation times, as well as provide full-gene phasing.

The presence of antibodies directed against HLA molecules expressed on the donor's cells is one the most important risk factor for serious clinical complications after transplantation. The lymphocyte crossmatch is one of the most important tests available to the laboratory as this assay detects the presence of donor-specific anti-HLA antibodies in potential allograft recipients. Early crossmatch methods used a complement-dependent cytotoxicity test, which was useful for detecting anti-HLA antibodies responsible for hyperacute graft rejection but lacked adequate sensitivity and specificity. Consequently, more sensitive and specific crossmatch methods were developed ultimately leading to the flow cytometry crossmatch as the preferred methodology.

HLA epitope matching provides a better approach to stratify patients at risk of developing antibody-mediated rejection compared with counting HLA mismatches. However, several immunologic parameters are not incorporated into these algorithms used to assess HLA epitopes, raising questions about the predictive value of these programs. Therefore, it is imperative to obtain more 3D structural data of antibody-antigen binding to "train" these computer algorithms. Also, mechanistic studies should be performed to prove these theoretic "epitopes." Most important, more information is needed to ensure these predictive computer algorithms are equitable and safe to use in clinical diagnostics before wide-scale implementation.

Advances in posttransplant care, including new immunosuppressive medications have led to excellent short-term renal allograft survival. However,
there is a small therapeutic window within which the patient and the clinician must balance the risk of rejection, with side effects such as infection,
malignancy, and toxicity. Laboratory testing plays a key role in this ongoing
monitoring, which includes relatively simple tests, such as serum creatinine, to complex tests, such as solid-phase assays, used to monitor for
donor-specific antibody and surveillance allograft biopsies. This article reviews the role of the laboratory tests and surveillance biopsies in posttransplant monitoring.

Conventional assessment of renal transplant rejection and injury through
use of histology, C4d staining, and HLA antibody testing, has been the
standard approach to transplant management. By many measures, these
methods of conventional assessment may be considered flawed, particularly with the subjective nature of histologic diagnoses. The Alberta Transplant Applied Genomics Center has developed the Molecular Microscope
diagnostic system, which uses microarrays to measure gene expression.
These data are analyzed using classifiers (weighted equations) that
compare the tested biopsy to a proprietary reference set of biopsies to
provide objective measures of the status of the renal transplant.

Natural killer (NK) cells use variable inhibitory and activating killer cell
immunoglobulin-like receptors (KIR) to detect and eliminate virally-
infected or tumor-transformed cells. The effector function of a given NK
cell depends upon its KIR receptor-repertoire, HLA ligands used for
licensing at the time of its development, and ligands it senses on the targets. Genes encoding KIRs and HLA ligands are located on different
chromosomes, and feature substantial variations. Independent segregation of these genes results in variable KIR-HLA inheritance that would
contribute to the individual's immunity. This review describes KIR-HLA diversity and summarizes current knowledge on their implication in disease
associations.

Celiac disease is an autoimmune disease affecting the small intestine, triggered by gluten sensitization in genetically susceptible individuals worldwide. Celiac disease development is strongly linked to the presence of
HLA-DQ2 and/or DQ8, which present the immunogenic gluten peptides
and trigger the immune response leading to pathogenesis. Because of

the variability of clinical symptoms, the disease is often underdiagnosed. Intestinal biopsy and the presence of antibodies to deamidated gliadin and tissue transglutaminase are recommended diagnostic tools. Genetic testing for HLA DQ2 and DQ8 can be used to rule out disease in at-risk populations.

Severe adverse drug reactions are a common cause of morbidity and mortality. Some of the most severe reactions are immunologically mediated and have been linked to specific HLA alleles. The mechanisms underlying HLA-associated drug hypersensitivity are complex and not fully understood. Recent findings have provided insight into recognition mechanisms underlying drug-induced immunopathogenesis and criteria for increasing positive prediction of hypersensitivity. Refining pharmocogenetic testing strategies to better identify at-risk individuals can improve hypersensitivity prevention and mechanism characterization.

HLA molecules play a significant role in immunity and disease susceptibility. GWAS studies underline the critical role of the MHC region in a wide range of diseases and remind us that the HLA genes, included within the MHC, interact extensively with other genomic regions which influence their functions. Recently, MHC/HLA genomic sequences encoding for miRNAs have been reported to interact with targets within and outside the MHC, influencing the expression of many transcripts. High throughput sequencing technologies provide unique opportunities for complete HLA/MHC sequence characterization, helping to elucidate their interactive relationships in a plethora of physiological and disease processes.

CLINICS IN LABORATORY MEDICINE

Preface

HLA in Transplantation and Beyond

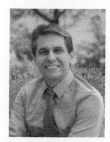 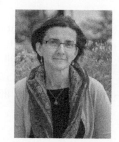

Julio C. Delgado, MD, MS   Eszter Lázár-Molnár, PhD
Editors

The HLA system consists of a very polymorphic set of genes, which are instrumental in orchestrating antigen-specific immune responses. This issue of *Clinics in Laboratory Medicine* is devoted to provide an overview of the importance of HLA in clinical diagnostics. The articles contributed by experts in the field focus on relevant areas ranging from transplantation testing to recent developments in HLA and disease associations. At the time of writing this preface, the total number of assigned HLA class I and class II alleles is over 20,000. This number is expected to grow rapidly due to recent advancements in HLA typing technologies and by adopting next-generation sequencing (NGS) in clinical HLA typing. Due to the significant impact of new technologies in the field, a review of the issue by Profaizer and Kumánovics discusses the opportunities and challenges of NGS-based HLA-typing platforms, which have revolutionized the field of HLA testing. Focusing on the role of HLA testing in transplantation, a technology-based article by Jaramillo, Ramon, and Stoll provides an overview of cross-matching in solid organ transplantation, followed by a review by Cusick and Jindra, discussing the opportunities and challenges of HLA epitope matching and its clinical applicability in donor selection for kidney transplantation.

The next two reviews of the special issue focus on recent advancements in monitoring the health and longevity of the transplanted organ. The Schinstock and Gandhi article discusses traditional serologic and histologic posttransplant monitoring approaches, followed by an article by Barner and colleagues describing a recently developed microarray-based molecular diagnostic test for renal transplant monitoring.

Consistent with its instrumental role in immune mechanisms, HLA has been recognized as an important genetic locus for disease susceptibility and drug hypersensitivity reactions. Several reviews are focused on this important topic; one of them by Raja discusses the interplay between HLA molecules and killer cell immunoglobulin-like receptors, followed by an article by Lázár-Molnár and Snyder about the role of HLA in

Clin Lab Med 38 (2018) xi–xii
https://doi.org/10.1016/j.cll.2018.10.001
0272-2712/18/© 2018 Published by Elsevier Inc.

labmed.theclinics.com

clinical diagnostic workup of celiac disease. A review by Ostrov discusses the significance of HLA testing in predicting drug hypersensitivity reactions. Finally, a review of the special issue by Shieh, Chitnis, and Monos addresses a broader perspective of HLA disease association in the context of developing technologies, which allow for the opportunity of dissecting interactions of HLA with other genomic regions, therefore proposing additional and possibly still unknown roles for HLA in health and disease.

Julio C. Delgado, MD, MS
University of Utah
ARUP Laboratories
500 Chipeta Way
Salt Lake City, UT 84108, USA

Eszter Lázár-Molnár, PhD
Histocompatibility & Immunogenetics Laboratory
University of Utah
ARUP Laboratories
500 Chipeta Way
Salt Lake City, UT 84108, USA

E-mail addresses:
julio.delgado@path.utah.edu (J.C. Delgado)
eszter.lazar-molnar@path.utah.edu (E. Lázár-Molnár)

Human Leukocyte Antigen Typing by Next-Generation Sequencing

Tracie Profaizer, MS*, Attila Kumánovics, MD

KEYWORDS

- Human leukocyte antigen (HLA) • Next generation sequencing (NGS)
- DNA sequencing • Polymerase chain reaction (PCR)

KEY POINTS

- HLA allele ambiguities are the result of limitations of current genotyping methodologies.
- Current next-generation sequencing (or second-generation sequencing) is superior to traditional technologies for high resolution HLA genotyping.
- Third-generation sequencing technologies in development offer the promise of phasing across the length of each HLA locus.

INTRODUCTION

The usefulness of HLA genotyping in solid organ and hematopoietic stem cell transplantation has been well-established.[1,2] Early HLA typing consisted of low-resolution or antigen-level assignments, but high-resolution genotyping has been shown to be important for the success of hematopoietic stem cell transplantation.[3] Furthermore, the identification of allele-specific antibodies suggests there are benefits to using high-resolution genotyping in solid organ transplantation as well, because it can more readily identify donors for highly sensitized transplant candidates.[4] HLA genotyping is also used for performing disease association testing because more than 100 diseases, including diabetes, rheumatoid arthritis, psoriasis, asthma, celiac disease, and narcolepsy, have been linked to various HLA alleles.[5] Associations with infectious diseases have also been identified and include human immunodeficiency virus infection, hepatitis, and tuberculosis, to list a few.[6] Moreover, drug reactions, such as Stevens-Johnson syndrome and toxic epidermal necrolysis, have been linked with certain medications and HLA allele combinations. Some of the most notable combinations include abacavir and HLA-B*57:01, carbamazepine and B*15:02, and allopurinol and B*58:01.[7]

Disclosure: The authors have nothing to disclose.
ARUP Institute for Clinical and Experimental Pathology, Department of Pathology, University of Utah School of Medicine, 500 Chipeta Way, Salt Lake City, UT 84108, USA
* Corresponding author.
E-mail address: tracie.profaizer@aruplab.com

Allelic variation is a major characteristic of the HLA system. Currently, there are more than 17,000 alleles published in the ImMunoGeneTics database, but less than 10% have been fully sequenced from the 5′ untranslated region to the 3′ untranslated region.[8] This growing list of alleles challenges the resolution capabilities of traditional technologies such as sequence-specific primer, sequence-specific oligonucleotide probe, and real-time polymerase chain reaction (PCR) assays. Even more sophisticated sequenced-based genotyping methods, such as Sanger sequencing, are lacking, because only exons 2 and 3 (and sometimes 4) for class I and only exon 2 for class II are sequenced in clinical settings. As a result, any coding variants outside of the sequenced region are neglected, resulting in ambiguous allele calls. This is particularly serious in hematopoietic stem cell transplantation recipients if a variant outside of these regions causes a null allele. Additionally, limiting the sequencing to the coding region neglects any intronic or other noncoding polymorphisms that may lead to splicing defects or affect protein expression.

The second challenge of HLA genotyping is cis/trans polymorphism. In Sanger sequencing, both alleles are sequenced in one reaction together. Thus, it is difficult to determine if 2 variants detected are from the same chromosome (cis) or from opposite chromosome (trans). It is not uncommon after Sanger sequencing for additional testing to be required to resolve alleles owing to this issue. The use of group-specific primers and family studies results in additional work, cost, and delays reporting.

SEQUENCE-BASED TYPING TECHNOLOGIES

Sequenced-based typing technologies can be categorized as first, second, and third generation. Each sequencing methodology is characterized by successive improvements in chemistry and software.

First-Generation Sequencing

Sanger sequencing

The first sequence-based typing method to obtain widespread acceptance is the Sanger sequencing method.[9] It is based on the premise of chain-terminating dideoxynucleotides, which halt the incorporation of additional nucleotides (**Fig. 1**). A mixture

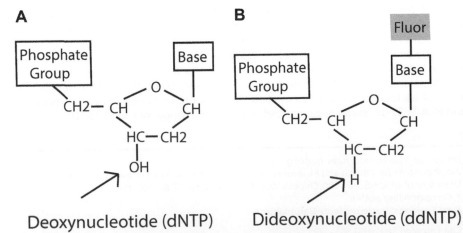

Fig. 1. Structures of nucleotides used in Sanger sequencing. Arrow points to site where incoming nucleotides can form a phosphodiester bond (*A*) or are terminated (*B*).

of the chain-terminating and fluorescently labeled chain-terminating dideoxynucleoti-des with regular nucleotides (dNTPs) yields sequenced fragments of varying sizes. Once the reaction is completed, the fragments are size separated on an agarose gel or by capillary electrophoresis. Shorter fragments migrate faster, with the largest fragments moving the slowest. The sequence can then be read from bottom to the top of the gel (or from the first-to-last reaching the end of capillaries) to determine the sequence. Although this method is robust and adequate for HLA typing, it has a number of shortcomings, including low throughput and high cost. Owing to its cost, it is only pragmatic to sequence the antigen recognition sites of class I and class II genes (exons 2–4 for class I and exon 2 for class II). Therefore, this method stills result in a number of allelic ambiguities. The highly polymorphic nature of HLA creates another problem, as discussed, which is the presence of cis/trans polymorphisms. This lack of phasing contributes to the number of ambiguities present.

Second-Generation Sequencing

Second-generation sequencing is known as next-generation sequencing (NGS) or massively parallel sequencing. The NGS process is often referred to as digital, because of the physical separation of the individual reactions.[10] Libraries of DNA are covalently attached to a solid support surface such as beads or slides (flow cells) before clonal amplification. Millions of individual sequencing reads is what makes this technology massive parallel sequencing. In contrast, the individual chain-terminating reactions in Sanger sequencing all take place in solution within the same reaction (analog).

Life Sciences/Roche 454

HLA genotyping using second-generation sequencing technology was first performed on the 454 Life Sciences (originally known as 454 Corporation, later acquired by Roche) Pyrosequencer (Roche, Basel, Switzerland), the first massively parallel sequencer to be commercially available.[11] The GS FLX and GS Junior are specific models of the 454 Pyrosequencer and both use the same chemistry. The 454 gener-ates clones of the same DNA library using emulsion PCR followed by pyrosequenc-ing.[12] The nucleotides used in pyrosequencing are not labeled. Rather, base detection occurs as the DNA polymerase adds incoming nucleotides to the growing strand releasing a pyrophosphate (**Fig. 2**A), initiating a reaction that results in the emis-sion of light.[13] To determine the correct order of bases, each of the 4 nucleotides must be added one at a time to the sequencing reaction to differentiate the signal.[14] In the event of a homopolymer (a string of the same bases), there are multiple successive in-corporations resulting in a higher signal intensity. Unfortunately, longer homopolymers may cause difficulties in accurately differentiating the number of bases, resulting in incorrect sequencing.[15] All of the early reports on HLA NGS were performed using the 454 technology, but Roche ended production of these sequencers in 2016.[16]

Roche Ion Torrent

Another sequencer produced by Thermo Fisher Scientific (Waltham, MA) for HLA gen-otyping is the Ion Torrent. Similar to the 454 Pyrosequencer, the chemistry is based on the use of emulsion PCR to generate clones of individual DNA libraries. But, rather than depending on a coupled reaction to generate a light signal, the Ion Torrent makes use of an integrated semiconductor and an ion-sensitive transistor to detect hydrogen ions as they are released each time a new nucleotide incorporated[14] (see **Fig. 2**A). Un-fortunately, the problems of the 454 are also found the Ion Torrent, namely, the pH change detected cannot always distinguish the length of homopolymer runs.

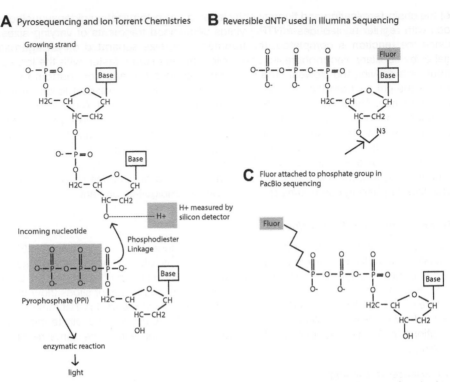

A Pyrosequencing and Ion Torrent Chemistries

B Reversible dNTP used in Illumina Sequencing

C Fluor attached to phosphate group in PacBio sequencing

Fig. 2. Next-generation sequencing. (*A*) Principle behind 454 and Ion Torrent chemistries. For the 454 pyrosequencing, incorporation of incoming nucleoside triphosphate releases pyrophosphate (PPi) which starts enzymatic reaction culminating in release of light. In Ion Torrent chemistry, the release of the hydrogen ion during incorporation is measured by a change in pH by the silicon detector. (*B*) Illumina chemistry. The 3′ group is a reversible blocked group (*arrow*). After incorporation and detection, the fluor and 3′blocked groups are cleaved and the 3′OH group is restored in preparation for the next nucleotide. (*C*) The PacBio makes use of a linker that attaches the fluor to the phosphate group of the incoming nucleotide. After incorporation, the fluor is cleaved eliminating a potential source of noise and steric hindrance.

Illumina sequencers (MiniSeq, MiSeq, NextSeq, HiSeq, and NovaSeq)

Illumina (San Diego, CA) offers a number of sequencers that vary in output, maximum reads per run, and read length.[17] Currently, the most popular sequencer for HLA genotyping is the Illumina MiSeq, which has gained widespread acceptance because of low error rates, including homopolymer regions of up to 9 base pairs in length.[18,19] Sequencing takes place on a solid surface, or flow cell, that is sealed and sandwiched between 2 glass slides. The flow cell is covered with a field of oligonucleotides, complementary to the adaptors that have been ligated to the DNA library. After attachment, the library undergoes an isothermal amplification to generate thousands of clonal copies or clusters of the same individual DNA fragment.[13] Because the ends of the DNA copies are available, universal sequencing primers are able to anneal and sequencing can begin. Illumina sequencing makes use of cyclic reversible termination chemistry.

The MiSeq has 4 imaging channels so that each of the 4 nucleotides will have its own spectrally unique fluorophore, but the other Illumina platforms only contain

2 imaging channels. For platforms with only 2 imaging channels, only C and T are labeled with a red and green fluorescent dye, respectively. When clusters are yellow, the nucleotide is identified as an A base. Clusters with no labeling are identified as a G base. By only using 2 channels, sequencing and data processing are faster and the optics are less expensive. Another unique feature of the newer Illumina sequencers is use of a patterned flow cell. Unlike the older Illumina flow cell, in which clusters can form anywhere on the surface of the flow cell, clusters can only generate in the distinct nanowells of the patterned flow cell. Because of the greater spatial separation, cluster identification is easier, data output is increased, and the run time is decreased. This process also makes the flow cell less susceptible to overloading.

An Illumina cycle starts with flooding the flow cell with the same nucleotide. After incorporation, the flow cell surface is imaged to determine which dNTP was added at each cluster. Next, the fluorophore is removed (**Fig. 2**B) and the 3' hydroxyl group is regenerated thus permitting continued DNA sequencing.[20]

Human Leukocyte Antigen Genotyping Considerations in Second-Generation Sequencing

Step 1: target preparation (targeted amplicon versus long-range polymerase chain reaction)

Nearly all of the early work in HLA genotyping started with only amplifying exons encoding the antigen recognition site.[21–24] Like Sanger sequencing, this approach neglects exons that do not code for the antigen recognition site or introns, so typing ambiguities will still be present. However, the benefits, compared with whole gene testing, include a shorter PCR time and an easier library preparation as these shorter amplicons do not need fragmentation.

The strategy that is becoming more widely accepted and practiced is the use of long-range PCR.[25] Even with the time required for long-range PCR, this approach can convey far more sequencing information than that provided by Sanger sequencing. Although long-range PCR of class I is relatively easy to design and perform, class II is more difficult because of its size and GC (guanine and cytosine) content. For example, DRB1 has a very large intron 1 (10,000 base pair) that is difficult to amplify. To overcome these difficulties, 2 primer sets can be used to amplify the desired gene or, alternatively, designing primers that skip intron 1 to amplify the gene starting with exon 2.

Preferential amplification is always a concern in any PCR-based protocol, especially for a polymorphic system such as HLA, which may lead to low coverage or dropouts for the poorly amplified allele.[26] This is particularly true with long-range PCR, where PCR efficiency decreases with increasing amplicon length. Therefore, it is crucial that allele balance be considered when analyzing the data, especially if 1 allele is significantly less represented than the other. It may indicate a poorly amplified allele or represent contamination. Importantly, a dropout allele may seemingly suggest that the sample is homozygous when it is not. In these situations, linkage disequilibrium and NGS sequencer quality metrics may be beneficial in identifying problems and suggesting further investigation. It is noteworthy that coamplification of nonclassical HLA genes (HLA-E, -F, -G, and -H) has been reported,[16] but these sequences can be bioinformatically removed.

Step 2: sequencing library preparation

Each of the second-generation sequencer platforms discussed have the following requirements after initial target generation (**Fig. 3**): cleaning and normalization of PCR

1. Generation of HLA amplicons by short or long-range PCR

1 A. If short-range (exon-based), can use primers that include instrument adaptors and unique indexes (not shown to scale):

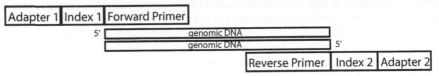

        -Amplicon clean-up and normalization
        -Pooling

1 B. If long-range, instrument adaptors and unique indexes are added post PCR:

        -Amplicon clean-up and normalization
        -Fragmentation
        -End-repair (blunt-ending and dA-tailing)

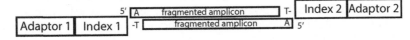

        -Pooling
        -Size selection
        -Clean-up

2. Final library quantification
3. Sequencer loading

Fig. 3. HLA next-generation sequencing (NGS) library preparation steps.

amplicons, a platform-specific sequencing library preparation, and then final library quantification before loading onto the sequencer. The differences in library preparation include whether short- or long-range PCR is used, when the instrument-specific adaptors and sample identification indices are ligated to the amplicons, and platform-specific sequencing requirements.

The efficiency and high-throughput capabilities of NGS depend on the ability to pool multiple samples and loci together in 1 sequencing reaction. Labeling individual samples and loci with unique DNA sequences may be known as molecular-barcoding, indexing, or multiplex identifiers (see **Fig. 3**). The early reports used fusion primers, which consisted of exon-specific primers, the 454 adaptor, and a sample DNA index or multiplex identifier.[21,22] The multiplex identifier was specific for each sample and exon used in the reaction; thus, each PCR amplicon was uniquely identified. When samples are indexed before PCR, pooling can take place immediately after amplicon clean-up and normalization, which simplifies library preparation.

However, this strategy only works when short amplicons are used. In the case of long-range PCR, indexing must take place after fragmentation and end repair. Only then can the instrument-specific adaptors and samples indices be added. Initially, there were questions concerning how to best index fragments generated from long-range PCR—by sample or by amplicon. In indexing by amplicon, each individual amplicon must be processed separately before any pooling can occur. This process adds more complexity to the library preparation process, but it also results in more reads per loci for analysis. A simpler approach is to pool the amplicons from each sample (indexing by sample) together after PCR and quantification so that each loci for each sample has the same index. This strategy only works if the bioinformatic software is sophisticated enough to obtain genotyping when cross-mapped reads from different loci may be present. Both approaches have been studied and compared, and several reports describe success with the index-by-sample strategy.[27,28] Improvements in software algorithms have now matured, and 11 loci from 1 patient can all be mixed in 1 tube after initial amplification and quantification. Regardless of the indexing strategy used, the advantage of multiplexing greatly simplifies the library preparation process[28] and pooling multiple patient samples together may lower the cost of high-resolution genotyping to less than traditional genotyping methodologies.[29]

Both the Illumina and Ion Torrent platforms use paired-end sequencing in which 2 sequencing reads are generated for every individual fragment, similar to the forward and reverse reads used in Sanger sequencing. For NGS, a forward, or read 1 and reverse, or read 2, are sequenced. This process doubles the amount of sequencing information available, which is useful for HLA genotyping, specifically, resolution of cis/trans polymorphisms. In NGS, typical sequenced read lengths are less than 300 base pairs, even though the actual DNA fragment size of the library may be larger. Through paired-end sequencing, both ends of the same fragment are sequenced, often leaving the middle unsequenced. This is not a drawback, but rather a useful tool because one long fragment can effectively anchor 2 distant polymorphisms to establish phasing. The average length of HLA antigen recognition site coding exons is 270 base pairs. Thus, polymorphisms that span exons and even into the introns can be phased. One study found that phasing polymorphisms 600 to 900 base pairs apart was most optimal.[28]

Regardless of the platform, the size of the DNA libraries is critical for successful NGS sequencing. Inserts that are too large will not clone and sequence as efficiently, but inserts that are too small will waste sequencing capacity and reagents. Another issue with small fragments is that the bioinformatic assembly of the short reads is harder and the phasing power is decreased in heterozygous samples.[30] Fragmentation of long-range amplicons to the desired size may be done enzymatically using endonucleases, physically using sonication, or by the use of transposons. Transposons-based methods are the most straightforward way to fragment because end-repair and adapter ligation occur simultaneously, decreasing time and sample handling; however, there is some evidence that transposon fragmentation is not truly random and GC bias is present, resulting in coverage loss and less sensitivity.[31] Physical fragmentation such as sonication is the most random way to accomplish fragmentation, but this method is less amenable to automation. Finally, in endonuclease digestion, 1 endonuclease will randomly nick a double-stranded DNA and another enzyme will recognize the nicked site and cut the opposite strand.[32] This method works well, but care must be taken when working with these enzymes to ensure that the correct incubation temperature and time are carefully adhered to prevent underfragmentation or overfragmentation.

Part of the library preparation process is the removal of fragments that are too short or long for reasons expressed herein. Therefore, a size separation method must be used to remove these unwanted fragments. This goal may be accomplished by gel electrophoresis, bead-based methods, or a size selection instrument. This step is also useful in removing library artifacts such as adapter dimers. These small fragments, if not removed, will take up valuable real estate on the flow cell or chip and do not generate any useful data.[33]

Final library quantification is important for optimal sequencing. For example, in the case of the MiSeq, overloading results in poor template generation and low sequencing owing to the clusters being too compacted. However, underloading wastes the flow cell and fewer data can be generated.[34] Generally, library quantitation can be done using a fluorometric measurement of DNA or more sensitively by real-time PCR. The advantage of using real-time PCR is that the primers are complementary to the instrument specific adaptors and, therefore, only adaptor-ligated libraries are quantified thereby providing useful information about the robustness of the library preparation process.

Step 3: bioinformatic analysis

A critical part of accurate HLA genotyping by NGS is the software used. Numerous software packages are available and all require the user to have a detailed knowledge of DNA alignment and mapping algorithms. Fortunately, the commercial HLA typing kits currently available come with user-friendly companion software that greatly simplifies the analysis process. Each option offers an array of quality control metrics to consider before final allele assignments are made. Some of the most important metrics are the QC30 score, read depth (or coverage), and allelic balance.

The probability of an incorrect base being called is known as a quality (Q) score and is related to error probability and is similar to the Phred quality score used in Sanger sequencing. Phred is a computer program that performs base calling and assigns an error probability to that base.[35,36] For NGS, the Q30 score is used as a metric and indicates that a base has a 1:1000 probability of being called incorrectly (or 99.9% base call accuracy).[37] The higher the Q30 score, the better the data.

Read depth (coverage) refers to the number of times an individual nucleotide is found in the final, aligned reads. Read depth directly impacts the sensitivity and specificity of the allele calls.[31,38] Moreover, the uniformity of coverage is very important so that all regions of both alleles are equally represented. Running fewer samples results in greater coverage per allele, but at a higher cost per sample. Conversely, running more samples means less coverage and possibly less confidence in the final result; therefore, a careful balance must be struck.[39]

Finally, allelic balance means that heterozygous alleles should be represented relatively equally among the sequence reads (approximately 50% each). When they are not, alleles may be erroneously assigned. Preferential amplification during PCR can lead to one allele being overamplified at the expense of the other as discussed in the Step 1: Target preparation (Targeted Amplicon vs Long-Range Polymerase Chain Traction) section. Examining the percentage of each allele can aid in assigning correct genotypes. Some groups recommend further investigation when allele imbalances are 30% to 70% or greater.[28]

Third-Generation Sequencing

Current NGS technologies are often called short read sequencing technologies because they are short as compared with Sanger sequencing, which can achieve sequencing results for around 1000 base pairs. They are also short compared with repetitive sequence domains seen in the human genome (eg, LINE and LTR genome-wide repeats), making bioinformatics difficult.[40] Third-generation technologies are long read sequencing that can achieve read lengths well beyond Sanger sequencing and overcome most problems caused by genome-wide repeats.[38] Third-generation sequencing technologies currently under development achieve long reads by interrogating the nucleotide sequences at the single molecule level in contrast to current NGS methods that require breaking long strands of DNA into smaller segments followed by clonal amplification. Hence, third-generation sequencing technologies are characterized by longer read lengths, a decrease in sequencing time, and a decrease in or elimination of sequencing biases introduced by PCR enrichment.[41] Library preparation requirements are minimal and, instead of relying on PCR to generate clusters, third-generation platforms can directly target single DNA molecules in real time so that the sequenced reads are ready for analysis immediately.[41] Both the Pacific Biosciences (Menlo Park, CA) and the Oxford Nanopore Technologies (Oxford, UK) MinION are in this category.[42]

Pacific Biosciences PacBio RS II

In second-generation sequencing, the sequence of a single molecule is derived from a cluster of clonally generated molecules, but the PacBio enables direct analysis of a single molecule meaning that no cluster generation is required.[43] This method reduces any bias introduced by PCR, which is important in a highly polymorphic system such as HLA. The PacBio RS II has 3 major advantages compared with second-generation platforms: long read lengths of greater than 30 kb, a low degree of bias (even across GC-rich regions), and the ability to detect DNA base modifications.[44,45] However, this technology still has some shortcomings, such as a high base calling error rate (>10%)[46] as well as a high rate of insertion or deletion errors, which create problems with homopolymers and repetitive sequences.[30] Despite these concerns, long read sequencing is desirable for HLA because it permits complete phasing across several kilobases of DNA. Furthermore, the types of errors seen with PacBio tend to be random and, with a sufficient sequencing depth, random errors can be discounted and discarded.[47]

The principle behind the PacBio RS II is based on a technology called zero-mode waveguides. The zero-mode waveguides are small holes, only tens of nanometers in diameter, and are smaller than the wavelength of the light used for detection. At the bottom of each hole, a single DNA polymerase is bound via biotin/streptavidin interaction. Each of the 4 nucleotides are uniquely labeled with a fluorophore and as they enter the zero-mode waveguide and fluoresce, only the bottom of the zero-mode waveguide is illuminated, causing only the nucleotide in the hole to fluoresce but not the ones above this bottom space. This is nonspecific because any nucleotide, incorporated or not, will fluoresce. Specificity occurs because the incorporation of the correct nucleotide takes milliseconds, approximately 3-fold longer than simple diffusion of nonincorporated nucleotides. The additional time taken by the correct nucleotide pairing creates a greater signal intensity than the background noise.[48] Another interesting feature of the PacBio RS II is that the fluorescent label is attached to the phosphate group, rather than the base, as in Illumina sequencing (**Fig. 2C**).[13] When, during the synthesis step, the phosphate group is cleaved off, so is the label, leaving the growing DNA chain ready to accept another new nucleotide.[48]

Oxford Nanopore MinION

The Nanopore MinION technology is based on the use of a modified hemolysin nanopore.[49] Through the hollow core of the bilayered lipid pore, single-stranded nucleic acid (DNA or RNA) is pulled through, one nucleotide at a time. Adaptors are ligated to both ends of the DNA, which permits capture of the DNA by the pore and subsequent loading of a processive enzyme at the 5' end. In this fashion, the nucleic acid moves through the pore unidirectionally. As each individual base moves through the pore, subtle differences in ionic current are detected by sensors with each base having its own unique ionic current signature.[50] An attractive feature of the MinION is its rapid turnaround time because of its ability to allow for real-time analysis as the DNA strands are translocated through the pore,[51] in contrast with the Illumina MiSeq run using standard 2 × 150-bp sequencing, which takes 20 hours in addition to the library preparation time. It was recently reported that the detection of the viral pathogens chikungunya virus, Ebola virus, and hepatitis C virus from human blood samples was accomplished in less than 6 hours of the initial sample acquisition.[52] If this technology translates to the HLA laboratory, it may allow for sequencing-based genotyping of deceased donors, which is not an option with the current sequencing methodologies.

Like the PacBio, the MinION can sequence long read lengths and simplify library preparation because no amplicon fragmentation is required. A recent report detailing the sequencing of a human reference genome found that they were able to obtain ultralong reads up to 882 kb in length.[53] Through use of these ultralong reads this study succeeded in the complete phasing of the entire 4-Mb major histocompatibility complex region, a feat not possible with second-generation platforms. It has been reported that error rates have a 92% read accuracy, suggesting that this technology is not quite ready for single nucleotide variant calling.[51] The sequencing errors can be attributed to 2 main problems. As stated elsewhere in this article, processive enzymes guide the DNA through the pore. Despite optimization the interval may fluctuate between the unidirectional migration of DNA from one nucleotide to the next inside the pore. If the interval is too short, bases maybe overlooked and missed. Too long of an interval and a single nucleotide may be denoted as a repetitive sequence. The other problem is due to the physical characteristic of the pore. It has been observed that up the 5 neighboring bases on the template DNA strand may simultaneously affect ionic current levels in the current instruments.[54] This problem has been largely addressed by software, but, ideally, the discovery of a different biological pore may ultimately solve this problem. Recently, experimental work using a single layer of graphene to create a pore suggests a possible solution.[55]

SUMMARY

NGS is a disruptive technology that is now rapidly becoming the new gold standard for high-resolution HLA typing. One important feature is its ability to generate more complete and better quality high-resolution genotyping data at a price comparable with or less expensive than traditional methods. Using NGS, additional typing technologies will no longer need to be performed to achieve high-resolution genotyping at the first pass, eliminating the need for reflexive testing. It is also disruptive because it changes the way histocompatibility laboratories operate. It was unheard of in the histocompatibility laboratory to mix multiple samples together, but with the advent and success of molecular bar coding, laboratories can decrease costs and still provide high-quality data. Commercially available HLA NGS genotyping kits with companion software make this technology now readily available to HLA laboratories. However, many challenges lie ahead. One is to make sense of the significance of coding and noncoding variants that are outside of the antigen recognition site. Other challenges include determining the optimal number of reporting fields to disclose to clinicians as well as establishing clinically relevant variants. Additional bioinformatic challenges await as new alleles are found daily.[56,57] The ImMunoGeneTics database will become even more useful as all the alleles can be fully sequenced. Finally, these new technologies can expand our knowledge beyond the HLA into the extended major histocompatibility complex to reveal relationships about disease and the immune system.[58,59]

REFERENCES

1. Petersdorf EW, Hansen JA, Martin PJ, et al. Major-histocompatibility-complex class I alleles and antigens in hematopoietic-cell transplantation. N Engl J Med 2001;345(25):1794–800.
2. Opelz G, Wujciak T, Dohler B, et al. HLA compatibility and organ transplant survival. Collaborative Transplant Study. Rev Immunogenet 1999;1(3):334–42.
3. Lee SJ, Klein J, Haagenson M, et al. High-resolution donor-recipient HLA matching contributes to the success of unrelated donor marrow transplantation. Blood 2007;2007(110):4576–83.
4. Duquesnoy RJ, Kamoun M, Baxter-Lowe LA, et al. Should HLA mismatch acceptability for sensitized transplant candidates be determined at the high-resolution rather than the antigen level? Am J Transplant 2015;15(4):923–30.
5. Trowsdale J, Knight JC. Major histocompatibility complex genomics and human disease. Annu Rev Genomics Hum Genet 2013;14:301–23.
6. Blackwell JM, Jamieson SE, Burgner D. HLA and infectious diseases. Clin Microbiol Rev 2009;22(2):370–85.
7. Negrini S, Becquemont L. HLA-associated drug hypersensitivity and the prediction of adverse drug reactions. Pharmacogenomics 2017;18(15):1441–57.
8. Robinson J, Halliwell JA, Hayhurst JD, et al. The IPD and IMGT/HLA database: allele variant databases. Nucleic Acids Res 2015;43(Database issue):D423–31.
9. Sanger F, Nicklen S, Coulson AR. DNA sequencing with chain-terminating inhibitors. Proc Natl Acad Sci U S A 1977;74(12):5463–7.
10. Mardis ER. Next-generation sequencing platforms. Annu Rev Anal Chem (Palo Alto Calif) 2013;6:287–303.
11. Hutchison CA 3rd. DNA sequencing: bench to bedside and beyond. Nucleic Acids Res 2007;35(18):6227–37.
12. Mardis ER. Next-generation DNA sequencing methods. Annu Rev Genomics Hum Genet 2008;9:387–402.
13. Metzker ML. Sequencing technologies - the next generation. Nat Rev Genet 2010;11(1):31–46.
14. Goodwin S, McPherson JD, McCombie WR. Coming of age: ten years of next-generation sequencing technologies. Nat Rev Genet 2016;17(6):333–51.
15. Shendure J, Ji H. Next-generation DNA sequencing. Nat Biotechnol 2008;26(10):1135–45.
16. Gabriel C, Furst D, Fae I, et al. HLA typing by next-generation sequencing - getting closer to reality. Tissue Antigens 2014;83(2):65–75.
17. Illumina. Illumina sequencing platforms. Description of Illumina sequencers. 2018. Available at: https://www.illumina.com/systems/sequencing-platforms.html. Accessed April 26, 2018.
18. De Santis D, Dinauer D, Duke J, et al. 16(th) IHIW: review of HLA typing by NGS. Int J Immunogenet 2013;40(1):72–6.
19. Duke JL, Lind C, Mackiewicz K, et al. Towards allele-level human leucocyte antigens genotyping – assessing two next-generation sequencing platforms: Ion Torrent Personal Genome Machine and Illumina MiSeq. Int J Immunogenet 2015;42(5):346–58.

20. Bentley DR, Balasubramanian S, Swerdlow HP, et al. Accurate whole human genome sequencing using reversible terminator chemistry. Nature 2008; 456(7218):53–9.
21. Bentley G, Higuchi R, Hoglund B, et al. High-resolution, high-throughput HLA genotyping by next-generation sequencing. Tissue Antigens 2009;74(5): 393–403.
22. Gabriel C, Danzer M, Hackl C, et al. Rapid high-throughput human leukocyte antigen typing by massively parallel pyrosequencing for high-resolution allele identification. Hum Immunol 2009;70(11):960–4.
23. Erlich RL, Jia X, Anderson S, et al. Next-generation sequencing for HLA typing of class I loci. BMC Genomics 2011;12:42.
24. Holcomb CL, Hoglund B, Anderson MW, et al. A multi-site study using high-resolution HLA genotyping by next generation sequencing. Tissue Antigens 2011;77(3):206–17.
25. Lind C, Ferriola D, Mackiewicz K, et al. Next-generation sequencing: the solution for high-resolution, unambiguous human leukocyte antigen typing. Hum Immunol 2010;71(10):1033–42.
26. Walsh PS, Erlich HA, Higuchi R. Preferential PCR amplification of alleles: mechanisms and solutions. PCR Methods Appl 1992;1(4):241–50.
27. Profaizer T, Coonrod EM, Delgado JC, et al. Report on the effects of fragment size, indexing, and read length on HLA sequencing on the Illumina MiSeq. Hum Immunol 2015;76(12):897–902.
28. Duke JL, Lind C, Mackiewicz K, et al. Determining performance characteristics of an NGS-based HLA typing method for clinical applications. HLA 2016;87(3): 141–52.
29. Weimer ET, Montgomery M, Petraroia R, et al. Performance characteristics and validation of next-generation sequencing for human leucocyte antigen typing. J Mol Diagn 2016;18(5):668–75.
30. Albrecht V, Zweiniger C, Surendranath V, et al. Dual redundant sequencing strategy: full-length gene characterisation of 1056 novel and confirmatory HLA alleles. HLA 2017;90(2):79–87.
31. Lan JH, Yin Y, Reed EF, et al. Impact of three Illumina library construction methods on GC bias and HLA genotype calling. Hum Immunol 2015;76(2–3): 166–75.
32. Voelkerding KV, Dames S, Durtschi JD. Next generation sequencing for clinical diagnostics-principles and application to targeted resequencing for hypertrophic cardiomyopathy: a paper from the 2009 William Beaumont Hospital Symposium on Molecular Pathology. J Mol Diagn 2010;12(5):539–51.
33. Head SR, Komori HK, LaMere SA, et al. Library construction for next-generation sequencing: overviews and challenges. Biotechniques 2014;56(2): 61–4, 66, 68.
34. Illumina. Diagnosing and preventing flow cell overclustering on the MiSeq system. 2015. Available at: https://support.illumina.com/content/dam/illumina-marketing/documents/products/other/miseq-overclustering-primer-770-2014-038.pdf. Accessed December 24, 2015.
35. Ewing B, Hillier L, Wendl MC, et al. Base-calling of automated sequencer traces using Phred. I. Accuracy assessment. Genome Res 1998;8(3):175–85.
36. Ewing B, Green P. Base-calling of automated sequencer traces using Phred. II. Error probabilities. Genome Res 1998;8(3):186–94.
37. Coonrod EM, Durtschi JD, Margraf RL, et al. Developing genome and exome sequencing for candidate gene identification in inherited disorders: an integrated

technical and bioinformatics approach. Arch Pathol Lab Med 2013;137(3): 415–33.

38. Sims D, Sudbery I, Ilott NE, et al. Sequencing depth and coverage: key considerations in genomic analyses. Nat Rev Genet 2014;15(2):121–32.

39. Sampson J, Jacobs K, Yeager M, et al. Efficient study design for next generation sequencing. Genet Epidemiol 2011;35(4):269–77.

40. Lander ES, Linton LM, Birren B, et al. Initial sequencing and analysis of the human genome. Nature 2001;409(6822):860–921.

41. Lu H, Giordano F, Ning Z. Oxford nanopore MinION sequencing and genome assembly. Genomics Proteomics Bioinformatics 2016;14(5):265–79.

42. Heather JM, Chain B. The sequence of sequencers: the history of sequencing DNA. Genomics 2016;107(1):1–8.

43. Erlich HA. HLA typing using next generation sequencing: an overview. Hum Immunol 2015;76(12):887–90.

44. Nakano K, Shiroma A, Shimoji M, et al. Advantages of genome sequencing by long-read sequencer using SMRT technology in medical area. Hum Cell 2017; 30(3):149–61.

45. Mardis ER. DNA sequencing technologies: 2006-2016. Nat Protoc 2017;12(2): 213–8.

46. Quail MA, Smith M, Coupland P, et al. A tale of three next generation sequencing platforms: comparison of Ion Torrent, Pacific Biosciences and Illumina MiSeq sequencers. BMC Genomics 2012;13:341.

47. Turner TR, Hayhurst JD, Hayward DR, et al. Single molecule real-time DNA sequencing of HLA genes at ultra-high resolution from 126 International HLA and Immunogenetics Workshop cell lines. HLA 2018;91(2):88–101.

48. Schadt EE, Turner S, Kasarskis A. A window into third-generation sequencing. Hum Mol Genet 2010;19(R2):R227–40.

49. Clarke J, Wu HC, Jayasinghe L, et al. Continuous base identification for single-molecule nanopore DNA sequencing. Nat Nanotechnol 2009;4(4):265–70.

50. Deamer D, Akeson M, Branton D. Three decades of nanopore sequencing. Nat Biotechnol 2016;34(5):518–24.

51. Jain M, Olsen HE, Paten B, et al. The Oxford Nanopore MinION: delivery of nanopore sequencing to the genomics community. Genome Biol 2016;17(1): 239.

52. Greninger AL, Naccache SN, Federman S, et al. Rapid metagenomic identification of viral pathogens in clinical samples by real-time nanopore sequencing analysis. Genome Med 2015;7:99.

53. Jain M, Koren S, Miga KH, et al. Nanopore sequencing and assembly of a human genome with ultra-long reads. Nat Biotechnol 2018;36(4):338–45.

54. Manrao EA, Derrington IM, Laszlo AH, et al. Reading DNA at single-nucleotide resolution with a mutant MspA nanopore and phi29 DNA polymerase. Nat Biotechnol 2012;30(4):349–53.

55. Garaj S, Liu S, Golovchenko JA, et al. Molecule-hugging graphene nanopores. Proc Natl Acad Sci U S A 2013;110(30):12192–6.

56. Milius RP, Heuer M, Valiga D, et al. Histoimmunogenetics markup language 1.0: reporting next generation sequencing-based HLA and KIR genotyping. Hum Immunol 2015;76(12):963–74.

57. Mack SJ, Milius RP, Gifford BD, et al. Minimum information for reporting next generation sequence genotyping (MIRING): guidelines for reporting HLA and KIR genotyping via next generation sequencing. Hum Immunol 2015;76(12): 954–62.

58. Hosomichi K, Shiina T, Tajima A, et al. The impact of next-generation sequencing technologies on HLA research. J Hum Genet 2015;60(11):665–73.
59. Clark PM, Kunkel M, Monos DS. The dichotomy between disease phenotype databases and the implications for understanding complex diseases involving the major histocompatibility complex. Int J Immunogenet 2015;42(6):413–22.

Technical Aspects of Crossmatching in Transplantation

Andrés Jaramillo, PhD*, Daniel S. Ramon, PhD, Scott T. Stoll, BS

KEYWORDS

- Complement-dependent cytotoxicity • Crossmatch
- Donor-specific anti-HLA antibody • Flow cytometry • Histocompatibility
- Anti-HLA antibody • Lymphocyte • Transplantation

KEY POINTS

- The presence of anti-HLA antibodies is one the most critical risk factors for serious clinical complications posttransplantation.
- The lymphocyte crossmatch is currently the only cell-based compatibility assay performed in most histocompatibility laboratories.
- The pioneer complement-dependent cytotoxicity crossmatch, introduced in the 1960s, was useful for detecting most anti-HLA antibodies that were responsible for hyperacute graft rejection but it lacked sufficient sensitivity to adequately guard against other types of antibody-mediated rejection.
- The flow cytometry crossmatch, introduced in the 1980s, is currently the most sensitive and reliable method for detecting anti-HLA antibodies that could lead to early graft loss posttransplantation.
- There are multiple technical factors to consider that significantly affect the sensitivity and specificity of the lymphocyte crossmatch.

INTRODUCTION

Two of the most important immunologic barriers in organ transplantation are ABO blood group incompatibility and the presence of anti-HLA antibodies in potential allograft recipients. The presence of antibodies directed against HLA molecules expressed on the donor's cells is a serious risk factor for clinical complications after transplantation. Depending on the strength of the donor-specific anti-HLA antibodies (DSA), the clinical impact may range from benign events, controlled with standard immunosuppression, to severe complications including graft loss.[1–3]

Disclosure Statement: This study was supported, in part, by a grant from the Mayo Clinic (A.J).
Histocompatibility Laboratory, Department of Laboratory Medicine and Pathology, Mayo Clinic, 5777 East Mayo Boulevard, Phoenix, AZ 85054, USA
* Corresponding author.
E-mail address: Jaramillo.Andres@mayo.edu

Regardless of the level of HLA matching, the most important test used in the laboratory is the lymphocyte crossmatch. This simple test assesses the level of DSA present in potential allograft recipients. Early crossmatch methods used a complement-dependent cytotoxicity (CDC) test, which was adequate for detecting most anti-HLA antibodies that were responsible for hyperacute graft rejection. However, this method did not detect low DSA levels that led to accelerated graft rejection and early graft loss. Consequently, more sensitive crossmatch methods were developed ultimately leading to the flow cytometry crossmatch (FCXM) as the preferred methodology. In this article, the authors review the evolution of the lymphocyte crossmatch assay and the important factors to take into consideration while performing, and interpreting results, of this fundamental assay for the fate of the transplanted organ.[4–7]

COMPLEMENT-DEPENDENT CYTOTOXICITY CROSSMATCH

The CDC crossmatch (CDCXM) was introduced in 1969 in a landmark paper that demonstrated for the first time that recipients with a positive crossmatch at the time of transplantation had significantly higher rates of hyperacute rejection.[8] Thus, the CDCXM immediately became the "gold standard" assay for the detection of DSA before transplantation. A significant reduction in hyperacute rejection rates was observed after implementing the requirement of a negative CDCXM before transplantation.[8,9]

The CDCXM is a biological assay that requires antibody binding, complement activation, and cellular damage to yield a positive reaction. Lymphocytes from the donor are first incubated with the patient's serum, followed by the addition of rabbit serum as a source of complement. If antibodies in the serum recognize HLA molecules expressed on the cells, activation of the complement cascade is initiated, leading to the assembly of the membrane attack complex on the plasmatic membrane and cell death. Percent cell death is determined by either the exclusion of a vital dye such as trypan blue or eosin or the uptake of a DNA staining fluorescent dye, such as ethidium bromide. The results are scored using a standardized ranking system based on the percentage of dead cells.[10–12] Although a significant improvement over the absence of any compatibility testing, the CDCXM had significantly high rates of false-negative and false-positive results. Thus, it lacked the sensitivity to detect all relevant alloantibodies and was unnecessarily excluding patients from transplants due to false-positive results.[13–15]

In an attempt to address some of the problems of the CDCXM, several modifications to the original method have been introduced. Such modifications included additional washes, extended incubations, and the addition of an anti-human globulin (AHG) to increase the sensitivity of the assay. In this regard, the most widely used modification to the CDCXM was the introduction of AHG in 1972 to augment the complement fixing ability of the sample.[16] AHG, a complement fixing antibody against human immunoglobulin, added as a second step, binds to any antibody bound to the target cells (both complement-binding and non-complement-binding antibodies), thereby increasing the antibody density, the likelihood of complement activation, and the sensitivity of the assay. Therefore, the AHG-augmented CDCXM rapidly emerged as a significant improvement over the standard CDCXM. This assay played a significant role in reducing early allograft rejection by detecting lower levels of anti-HLA antibodies and noncomplement fixing anti-HLA antibodies, referred to as cytotoxicity-negative, adsorption-positive (CYNAP) antibodies.[13,14,17] The anti-HLA antibodies detected by this method but not detected by the standard CDCXM were associated with higher rates of early allograft loss as compared with the ones observed in patients with a negative AHG-augmented CDCXM result.[15,17,18] Of note, both the standard and the AHG-augmented CDCXM can detect both immunoglobulin G (IgG) and IgM classes of antibodies. Although not considered clinically significant, IgM antibodies can interfere with the detection of IgG antibodies. Therefore, another common laboratory practice, aimed at increasing the specificity of the assay, is to pretreat the patient's serum with heat or a reducing agent, such as dithiothreitol, to break pentameric IgM into monomers, rendering them incapable of fixing complement.[17]

In conclusion, the CDCXM cannot detect anti-HLA antibodies that are either non-complement binding or at levels below the complement activation threshold. In addition, the CDCXM also displays a significant lack of sensitivity for detection of anti-HLA class II antibodies, which is not improved by AHG-augmentation due to nonspecific binding of AHG to Fc receptors on B cells.[19] Other disadvantages of the CDCXM include the difficulty to purify the large number of viable target cells necessary for testing, nonspecific cell death due to complement sensitivity that causes false-positive reactions, and the presence of anticomplementary factors in a patient's serum that can interfere with the efficacy of the assay and lead to a significantly high interlaboratory variability.[20] Although the AHG-augmented CDCXM represented an improvement over the standard CDCXM, it still suffers from the same problems intrinsic to the detection systems based on complement activation.[19,20]

FLOW CYTOMETRY CROSSMATCH

The original work from Patel and Terasaki[8] and several subsequent studies demonstrated that a significant number of patients with a negative CDCXM experienced early graft loss consistent with antibody-mediated rejection.[13–15,17,18,21] These findings suggested that low DSA levels, undetectable by the CDCXM, were present in the recipient at the time of transplantation. A significant improvement in sensitivity and specificity was achieved with the introduction of the FCXM in 1983.[22] This and other studies showed that the FCXM was capable of detecting low DSA levels not previously detected by the CDCXM.[22–25] Most notable, renal transplant recipients exhibiting negative CDCXM or AHG-augmented CDCXM but positive FCXM were more likely to experience early accelerated rejection episodes and graft loss.[26–29] Hence, the FCXM for the assessment of DSA reactivity quickly replaced the CDCXM as the standard pretransplant crossmatch test.

The FCXM is performed by incubating donor's cells with patient's serum. If DSA are present in the patient's serum, they will bind to HLA molecules expressed on the donor's cells. After washing away unbound antibodies and other serum components, assessment of DSA binding is performed by the addition of a fluorescein isothiocyanate (FITC)-conjugated anti-human IgG to detect DSA bound to the cells. The fluorescence intensity emitted is proportional to the amount of DSA bound to the cells. A subsequent refinement introduced 3-color flow cytometry to allow for the simultaneous assessment of T and B cell reactivities without physically separating the lymphocyte populations[24] (**Fig. 1**). This technique incorporated an additional incubation with peridinin-chlorophyll-protein (PerCP) complex-conjugated anti-CD3 and phycoerythrin (PE)-conjugated anti-CD19 monoclonal antibodies to identify the T and B cell populations, respectively. The 3-color FCXM allowed for the simultaneous detection of DSA reacting with T and B cells and eliminated background staining due to DSA binding to nonlymphocytic mononuclear cells. Postacquisition analysis then allowed for the independent evaluation of DSA reactivity to each cell population. Interpretation of the FCXM is performed by comparing the fluorescence intensity of the target cell population treated with patient's serum to the fluorescence intensity of

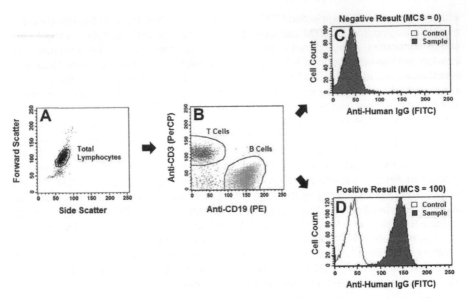

Fig. 1. Representative plots from a typical 3-color FCXM. (*A*) Forward scatter versus side scatter plot illustrating the gating of lymphocytes isolated by negative selection. (*B*) CD3 versus CD19 plot illustrating the ability to simultaneously identify T and B cell populations. (*C*) Overlay histogram of the negative control and a patient's serum showing a negative result. (*D*) Overlay histogram of the negative control and a patient's serum showing a positive result.

the same cell population treated with a negative control serum. Results are commonly reported as fluorescence median channel shifts (MCS) above the negative control serum. The interpretation of the FCXM is more objective than the visual assessment used in the CDCXM and has the added advantage of being semiquantitative in that the MCS value indicates the relative amount of DSA bound to the target cells.[4,5,23,24,30–32]

Even though the FCXM is currently the most sensitive crossmatch method available, it too suffers from many of the same problems associated with other cell-based assays.[19] Most notably, nonspecific immunoglobulin binding to Fc receptors, non-HLA autoantibodies, and therapeutic antibodies used for immunosuppressive induction therapy, such as rituximab (anti-CD20), daclizumab (anti-CD25), alemtuzumab (anti-CD52), and anti-thymocyte globulin, can all lead to false-positive FCXM results.[33–36]

VARIABLE EXPRESSION AND DISTRIBUTION OF HLA MOLECULES

It is important to mention that T cells express only HLA class I molecules, whereas B cells express higher levels of HLA class I as well as HLA class II molecules.[19,37–41] Because of this differential expression and distribution of HLA molecules on T and B cells, the 3-color FCXM provides, with some limitations, additional information about the DSA reactivity of the patient (HLA class I vs class II) (**Table 1**). HLA expression is also known to vary between HLA loci; it is higher for HLA-A, -B, and DRB1 as compared with HLA-C, DRB3/4/5, DQB1, and DPB1.[37–42] Expression also varies among different alleles within the same HLA locus,[43–45] and previous studies have indicated that HLA-C is expressed at higher levels on T cells as compared with B cells producing, in some instances, unusual positive T cell/negative B cell FCXM results

Table 1		
Flow cytometry crossmatch interpretation		
T Cell Reactivity	**B Cell Reactivity**	**Donor-Specific Anti-HLA Antibody**
Negative	Negative	None or low levels
Positive	*Positive*	HLA class I or HLA class I and II
Negative	*Positive*	HLA class II or low levels of HLA class I
Positive	Negative	Non-HLA autoantibody or HLA-C[a]

[a] Note: observed in selected cases.

(see **Table 1**).[46,47] Other studies have shown a significant variability of HLA expression on lymphocytes from different donor types (living or deceased) and from different tissues (peripheral blood, lymph node, or spleen).[48] It is also pertinent to consider that HLA expression is affected by extrinsic factors, such as age, infection, disease, and medications.[49–52]

TARGET CELL PREPARATION

The most common sources of target cells in the FCXM are mononuclear cells derived from peripheral blood, lymph node, or spleen. To this day, density gradient centrifugation is still used by many laboratories for mononuclear cell isolation. This procedure is labor-intensive and time-consuming, and depending on the age and quality of the sample, the mononuclear cell yield and purity display significant variation from donor to donor.[53] Furthermore, the purity of the lymphocyte population in mononuclear cell preparations enriched by density gradient centrifugation is low and highly variable with yields of less than 10% and 55% of lymphocytes (T and B cells) in spleen (**Fig. 2**A) and peripheral blood (**Fig. 2**B), respectively.[54] In contrast, lymphocyte isolation by negative selection using magnetic beads consistently yields more than 85% and 90% of purified lymphocytes (T and B cells) in spleen (see **Fig. 2**A) and peripheral blood (see **Fig. 2**B), respectively.[54] Poor lymphocyte purity has a considerable effect on the FCXM results because nonlymphocytic cells in the mononuclear cell preparation also express HLA molecules. Therefore, if the patient's serum contains low levels of DSA, these antibodies would be incorporated by both lymphocytes and nonlymphocytic cells reducing the total amount of antibody binding to the target cell population (lymphocytes) and potentially leading to a false-negative FCXM result.[23,53] On this matter, **Table 2** shows that the FCXM performed with the negative selection method displays significantly higher sensitivity than the FCXM performed with the density gradient centrifugation method.[54]

It is worth mentioning that the actual cell concentration is not critical for the outcome of the FCXM; however, the cell number is extremely important. The most crucial variable when performing the FCXM is the cell to serum ratio. Increasing the serum volume or decreasing the cell number will increase the sensitivity of the FCXM. On the contrary, decreasing the serum volume or increasing the cell number will significantly decrease the sensitivity of the FCXM.[54] **Fig. 3**A shows an FCXM performed with 1.25×10^5 cells with a serum containing low levels of DSA yielded a fluorescence intensity that was significantly higher than the fluorescence intensity observed in an FCXM performed with 10×10^5 cells.[54] These data show that the cell number is inversely proportional to the FCXM reactivity and may have a significant impact on the outcome of the FCXM, especially in patients showing weak DSA reactivity. Of note, a parallel FCXM performed at an optimal concentration of a monoclonal antibody directed against HLA class I molecules was not affected by the cell number (**Fig. 3**B).[54]

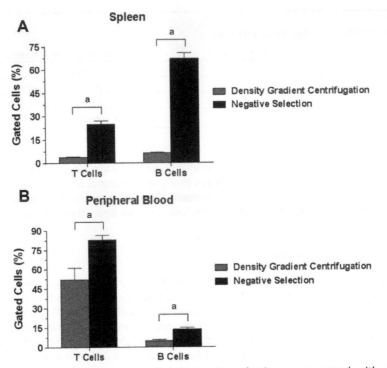

Fig. 2. Higher purity of T and B cells by negative selection as compared with density gradient centrifugation. Lymphocytes were isolated from spleen (n = 10) (A) or peripheral blood (n = 10) (B) by density gradient centrifugation or negative selection. Then, 2-color flow cytometry analysis of T and B cells was performed with PerCP-conjugated anti-CD3 and PE-conjugated anti-CD19 monoclonal antibodies, respectively. Results are expressed as the mean ± standard deviation. Differences in the percentage of gated T and B cells were analyzed by 2-tailed paired Student t test: [a] P<.01.

Table 2
Performance characteristics of the density gradient centrifugation method as compared with the negative selection method

| | T Cell FCXM (n = 20) | | B Cell FCXM (n = 20) | |
| | Density Gradient Centrifugation | | Density Gradient Centrifugation | |
	Positive	Negative	Positive	Negative
Negative Selection				
Positive	13	4	15	4
Negative	0	3	0	1
Sensitivity (95% CI)	76.4% (50.1%–93.2%)		79% (54.4%–94%)	
Specificity (95% CI)	100% (29.2%–100%)		100% (2.5%–100%)	
PPV (95% CI)	100% (75.3%–100%)		100% (78.2%–100%)	
NPV (95% CI)	42.9% (9.8%–81.6%)		20% (0.5%–71.6%)	
P value	.03		.25	

Abbreviations: CI, confidence interval; NPV, negative predictive value; PPV, positive predictive value.

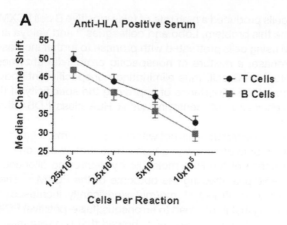

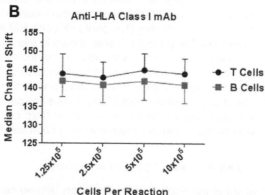

Fig. 3. Inverse correlation between cell number and FCXM reactivity. FCXM were performed with a serum containing low levels of DSA with a varying number of cells (1.25×10^5 to 10×10^5) (n = 5) (A). Qualitative assessment of HLA expression was determined by staining cells with a FITC-conjugated anti-HLA class I monoclonal antibody (clone W6/32) (n = 5) (B). Positive T and B cell FCXM reactivity represented MCS values greater than 20 and 30, respectively (0–256 scale). Results are expressed as the mean ± standard deviation. mAb, monoclonal antibody.

This result can be explained by the significantly higher affinity and saturating concentration of the monoclonal antibody used in this experiment that is seldom found in a patient's serum. The FCXM is a laboratory-developed test; thus, the cell number and serum volume used per reaction vary significantly among laboratories. Most laboratories use a cell number between 2.5×10^5 and 5×10^5 and a serum volume between 20 and 100 μL per reaction. Generally, a cell number that does not exceed 2.5×10^5 and a serum volume between 20 and 50 μL per reaction are recommended. Such heterogeneity explains the high interlaboratory variability of FCXM results.[25]

EFFECT OF PRONASE ON THE FLOW CYTOMETRY CROSSMATCH

As mentioned above, T cells express only HLA class I molecules, whereas B cells express both HLA class I and class II molecules.[19,37–41] Thus, the B cell FCXM was considered a more sensitive assay for evaluating transplant recipients.[19] However, nonspecific binding of immunoglobulins to the Fc and complement receptors expressed on B cells produced a high rate of false-positive B cell FCXM results.[19] In an effort to overcome this problem, Lobo and colleagues[55] and Vaidya and colleagues[56] performed FCXM using cells pretreated with pronase to further increase the specificity of the assay. Pronase, a mixture of nonspecific proteolytic enzymes, was used to cleave Fc receptors on B cell, thus eliminating nonspecific antibody binding. Their findings underscored the importance of improving the specificity of the B cell FCXM as well as the significance of identifying weak HLA class I DSA that are detected mainly on B cells.

Nevertheless, pronase treatment is not without its problems. It has been reported that extended incubation or treatment with a high concentration of pronase (2 mg/mL) may affect the conformation of the HLA molecule by destroying allogeneic epitopes and exposing cryptic epitopes affecting the outcome of the FCXM.[57] These studies also showed that pronase treatment (1 mg/mL) significantly increased reactivity of the T cell FCXM indicating that it may lead to erroneous (false-positive) FCXM results. Subsequent studies by Park and colleagues[58] showed that pronase treatment (1 mg/mL) induced 13.3% of false-positive T cell FCXM results. In this regard, Szewczyk and colleagues[36] showed that pronase treatment (1 mg/mL) induces 100% of false-positive T cell FCXM results in HIV-positive patients. It was shown in this study that the T cell FCXM reactivity with pronase-treated cells was induced by non-HLA autoantibodies. Overall, these data indicate that pronase treatment induces false-positive T cell FCXM results in selected groups of patients. Laboratories using pronase in their FCXM protocol should examine the rate of false-positive T cell FCXM results and consider testing these patients in parallel with nontreated cells to prevent them from being inappropriately excluded from receiving an organ due to a false-positive FCXM result.

SECONDARY ANTI-HUMAN IMMUNOGLOBULIN ANTIBODY

The most critical reagent of the FCXM is the secondary anti-human immunoglobulin antibody. This reagent is used to identify the antibody that is specifically bound to the cell. As such, this reagent should be selected to provide optimum sensitivity and specificity. Secondary antibodies can be selected that are specific for the various classes and subclasses of immunoglobulins. An optimal secondary antibody should display the following characteristics: (1) well-defined specificity (IgG or IgM), (2) contain only an F(ab')$_2$ fragment to reduce nonspecific binding to Fc receptors, and (3) display minimal cross-reactivity with immunoglobulins of other species. Currently, the most widely used secondary antibody is an FITC-conjugated F(ab')$_2$ goat anti-human IgG (Fc-specific) polyclonal antibody. Each lot of this secondary antibody requires extensive validation and should be titered to determine the optimum working dilution. Toward this, several dilutions of the secondary antibody are tested against T and B cells that have been preincubated with a well-defined positive control serum. Although higher fluorescence intensity may be observed with higher concentrations (lower dilutions) of the secondary antibody, a higher MCS value may be observed at lower concentrations (higher dilutions) of this reagent. Predominantly, this is the result of lower nonspecific binding of the secondary antibody at lower dilutions. There is a significant difference in the level of nonspecific binding among lots of secondary polyclonal antibody. Subsequently, it is difficult to find 2 lots that have comparable sensitivity and specificity.

Because of the difficulties mentioned above, the authors' laboratory opted to use an FITC-conjugated mouse anti-human IgG monoclonal antibody as secondary antibody for which the lot-to-lot variation is minimal.[54] As shown in **Table 3**, a comparison of the performance characteristics of the FCXM performed with polyclonal versus monoclonal secondary antibody shows that the FCXM performed with the monoclonal antibody displays significantly higher sensitivity and specificity than the FCXM performed with the polyclonal antibody.[54] These data indicate that the higher sensitivity and specificity observed with the monoclonal antibody is due to the inherently low nonspecific binding observed with this type of antibody.[59,60] The issue of cross-reactivity against immunoglobulins of other species is also nonexistent when using a monoclonal antibody and may contribute to its better performance. The secondary monoclonal antibody is more expensive than the polyclonal antibody, but the higher consistency between lots and the significantly higher sensitivity and specificity observed with this reagent makes it a more reliable reagent to use in the FCXM procedure.[54]

POSITIVE AND NEGATIVE CONTROLS

The FCXM requires both positive and negative control reagents. However, there are no commercial control reagents available specifically designed for the FCXM. Therefore, each laboratory must establish its own set of control reagents and positive cutoff values for the interpretation of the FCXM. The normal human serum used as negative control is the most important control reagent used in the FCXM. This reagent is usually obtained from a single or a pool of normal male donors known to be negative for anti-HLA antibodies. Serum from female donors may be used provided the donors have not had any pregnancies. The reason for this being that during pregnancy women are exposed to paternal HLA molecules and have the potential to be sensitized against these antigens. There are several commercially available normal human sera collected from large pools of normal blood group AB male donors that can be used as negative control. Nevertheless, a thorough screening of any potential negative control should be performed by means of FCXM using cells from different donors (n ≥5), solid-phase phenotype bead assays, and solid-phase single antigen bead assays to ensure that the reagent has no reactivity to lymphocytes and, more importantly, to HLA molecules.

To determine the normal range of fluorescence intensity obtained with the negative control, several FCXM should be performed using cells from individuals whose HLA types cover most of the HLA specificities (n ≥20). The fluorescence intensity for each FCXM should be recorded without changing any instrument settings. Then,

Table 3
Performance characteristics of the polyclonal antibody method as compared with the monoclonal antibody method

| | T Cell FCXM (n = 100) | | B Cell FCXM (n = 100) | |
| | Polyclonal Antibody | | Polyclonal Antibody | |
	Positive	Negative	Positive	Negative
Monoclonal Antibody				
Positive	70	4	59	26
Negative	2	24	1	14
Sensitivity (95% CI)	94.6% (86.7%–98.5%)		69.4% (58.5%–79%)	
Specificity (95% CI)	92.3% (74.9%–100%)		93.3% (69%–99.8%)	
PPV (95% CI)	97.2% (90.3%–99.7%)		98.3% (91.1%–100%)	
NPV (95% CI)	85.7% (67.3%–96.0%)		35% (20.6%–51.7%)	
P value	<.0001		<.0001	

a calculation of the mean and standard deviation of the fluorescence intensity for both T and B cell populations should be performed. Using 2 to 3 standard deviations (to cover 95.4% to 99.7% of the population), it is possible to define a cutoff value that can be used as a discriminator for positivity.[23] Thus, with a high degree of statistical confidence, an MCS value observed in a patient's serum that is greater than the chosen cutoff value between 2 to 3 standard deviations may be considered a positive result. The distinction between weakly positive and negative results is particularly problematic with the FCXM. For this reason, each laboratory must establish its own cutoff values to be used as discriminators for positivity. These cutoff values, however, are not absolute, and new cutoff values should be established with each new lot of negative control.

In contrast to the negative control, the positive control is easier to obtain. This reagent usually consists of pooled sera from of sensitized patients who are known to have high levels of anti-HLA antibodies, with a panel reactive antibody (PRA) greater than 80%, and whose combined antibody profile covers 100% of the HLA antigens. An undiluted positive control reagent will usually produce very strong positive results that are seldom observed with patient's serum. Therefore, when determining an appropriate working dilution, it is important to use the positive control at a dilution that yields a moderate to low fluorescence intensity (at non-saturating levels of DSA). In this regard, it is important to emphasize that the FCXM should be optimized for the detection of low levels of anti-HLA antibodies. Hence, using a positive control that exhibits a moderate to low fluorescence intensity will help in the daily assessment of the FCXM performance. For example, if the positive control regularly exhibits an MCS value of 80 to 100 when the cutoff value for a positive result is 20 to 30 MCS (0–256 scale), then an FCXM in which the positive control exhibits an MCS value of 40 to 50 may be an indication of an invalid test. Conversely, a strong positive control that normally yields an MCS value of 220 to 240 does not add any useful information. Significant errors could be made that would not necessarily result in a significant change of the fluorescence intensity of the positive control. Conversely, a lower working dilution of the positive control would be more sensitive to deviations in the system.

COMPARISON BETWEEN COMPLEMENT-DEPENDENT CYTOTOXICITY CROSSMATCH AND FLOW CYTOMETRY CROSSMATCH

Currently, most transplant centers considered the FCXM the "gold standard" for the detection of DSA. Indeed, it is well known that the FCXM is a more sensitive technique to detect DSA and is a better predictor of outcome in renal transplantation than the CDCXM.[8,9,13,15,17,18,21,23,61] However, to date, no direct analysis has been performed to determine the correlation between and the CDCXM outcome and the FCXM reactivity. Therefore, in order to determine a correlation between the CDCXM and the FCXM, the authors retrospectively performed an analysis of a large number of crossmatch pairs performed simultaneously by CDCXM and FCXM at a single laboratory. **Table 4** shows that the T and B cell CDCXM displayed a sensitivity of 34.7% and 40%, respectively, as compared with the FCXM. Furthermore, these data showed a linear correlation between the CDCXM outcome and the FCXM reactivity (**Fig. 4**A, B). Interestingly, less than 50% of the CDCXM were positive when the FCXM displayed an MCS value lower than 70 to 80. Even with a very strong MCS value greater than 100 observed, the percentage of positive T and B cell CDCXM results only reached 92% and 88%, respectively. These data showed the significantly lower sensitivity of the CDCXM as compared with the FCXM and also the ability of the FCXM to

Table 4
Performance characteristics of the complement-dependent cytotoxicity crossmatch as compared with flow cytometry crossmatch

| | T Cell (n = 30,303) | | B Cell (n = 27,686) | |
| | CDCXM | | CDCXM | |
	Positive	Negative	Positive	Negative
FCXM				
Positive	2968	*5580*	3297	*4939*
Negative	217	21,538	988	18,462
Sensitivity (95% CI)	*34.7% (33.7%–35.7%)*		*40% (39%–41.1%)*	
Specificity (95% CI)	99% (98.9%–99.1%)		94.9% (94.6%–95.2%)	
PPV (95% CI)	93.2% (92.3%–94%)		76.9% (75.7%–78.2%)	
NPV (95% CI)	79.4% (78.9%–79.9%)		78.9% (78.4%–79.4%)	
P value	<.0001		<.0001	

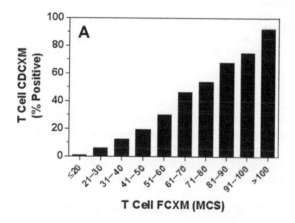

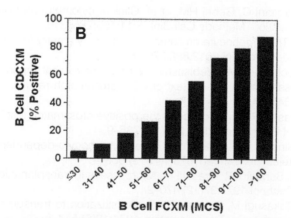

Fig. 4. Comparison between CDCXM and FCXM. T cell (n = 30,303) (*A*) and B cell (n = 27,686) (*B*) CDCXM and FCXM were performed in parallel at a single laboratory. Then, a comparison between the FCXM reactivity and the CDCXM outcome was performed by linear regression. Positive T and B cell FCXM reactivity represented MCS values greater than 20 and 30, respectively (0–256 scale).

detect a subset of noncomplement binding antibodies that may be clinically relevant after transplantation.

SUMMARY

The lymphocyte crossmatch is currently the only compatibility assay performed in most histocompatibility laboratories. The classical CDCXM was useful for detecting most anti-HLA antibodies responsible for hyperacute allograft rejection, but it lacked sufficient sensitivity to adequately guard against other types of antibody-mediated rejection. Advances in flow cytometry, molecular biology, and protein chemistry contributed to the development of the FCXM assay that has rapidly replaced the classical CDCXM and provides a more sensitive method for the final compatibility assessment before the transplant. In conjunction with the new solid-phase bead assays for anti-HLA antibody testing, the FCXM has contributed significantly to the understanding of the role of anti-HLA antibodies in the process of allograft rejection and to a significantly higher number of organ transplants with a greater degree of safety in sensitized individuals.

ACKNOWLEDGMENTS

This study was supported, in part, by a grant from the Mayo Clinic (A.J.).

REFERENCES

1. Lefaucheur C, Viglietti D, Mangiola M, et al. From humoral theory to performant risk stratification in kidney transplantation. J Immunol Res 2017;2017:5201098.
2. Mehra NK, Baranwal AK. Clinical and immunological relevance of antibodies in solid organ transplantation. Int J Immunogenet 2016;43(6):351–68.
3. Valenzuela NM, Reed EF. Antibody-mediated rejection across solid organ transplants: manifestations, mechanisms, and therapies. J Clin Invest 2017;127(7):2492–504.
4. Bray RA. Lymphocyte crossmatching by flow cytometry. Methods Mol Biol 2013;1034:285–96.
5. Bray RA, Tarsitani C, Gebel HM, et al. Clinical cytometry and progress in HLA antibody detection. Methods Cell Biol 2011;103:285–310.
6. Downing J. The lymphocyte crossmatch by flow cytometry for kidney transplantation. Methods Mol Biol 2012;882:379–90.
7. Graff RJ, Buchanan PM, Dzebisashvili N, et al. The clinical importance of flow cytometry crossmatch in the context of CDC crossmatch results. Transplant Proc 2010;42(9):3471–4.
8. Patel R, Terasaki PI. Significance of the positive crossmatch test in kidney transplantation. N Engl J Med 1969;280(14):735–9.
9. Stiller CR, Sinclair NR, Abrahams S, et al. Lymphocyte-dependent antibody and renal graft rejection. Lancet 1975;1(7913):953–4.
10. Takasugi M, Sengar DP, Terasaki PI. Microassays in transplantation immunology. Am J Med Technol 1971;37(12):470–2.
11. Tanaka N, Takasugi M, Terasaki PI. Presensitization to transplants detected by cellular immunity tests. Transplantation 1971;12(6):514–8.
12. Terasaki PI, McClelland JD. Microdroplet assay of human serum cytotoxins. Nature 1964;204:998–1000.
13. Amos DB, Cohen I, Klein WJ Jr. Mechanisms of immunologic enhancement. Transpl Proc 1970;2(1):68–75.

14. Fuller TC, Fuller AA, Golden M, et al. HLA alloantibodies and the mechanism of the antiglobulin-augmented lymphocytotoxicity procedure. Hum Immunol 1997; 56(1–2):94–105.

15. Kerman RH, Kimball PM, Van Buren CT, et al. Improved renal allograft survival for AHG and DTE/AHG crossmatch-negative recipients. Transpl Proc 1991;23(1 Pt 1):400–2.

16. Johnson AH, Rossen RD, Butler WT. Detection of alloantibodies using a sensitive antiglobulin microcytotoxicity test: identification of low levels of pre-formed antibodies in accelerated allograft rejection. Tissue Antigens 1972;2(3):215–26.

17. Kerman RH, Kimball PM, Van Buren CT, et al. AHG and DTE/AHG procedure identification of crossmatch-appropriate donor-recipient pairings that result in improved graft survival. Transplantation 1991;51(2):316–20.

18. Kerman RH. The role of crossmatching in organ transplantation. Arch Pathol Lab Med 1991;115(3):255–9.

19. Delgado JC, Eckels DD. Positive B-cell only flow cytometric crossmatch: implications for renal transplantation. Exp Mol Pathol 2008;85(1):59–63.

20. Duquesnoy RJ, Marrari M. Multilaboratory evaluation of serum analysis for HLA antibody and crossmatch reactivity by lymphocytotoxicity methods. Arch Pathol Lab Med 2003;127(2):149–56.

21. Cross DE, Whittier FC, Weaver P, et al. A comparison of the antiglobulin versus extended incubation time crossmatch: results in 223 renal transplants. Transplant Proc 1977;9(4):1803–6.

22. Garovoy MR, Rheinschmidt MA, Bigos M, et al. Flow cytometry analysis: a high technology crossmatch technique facilitating transplantation. Transplant Proc 1983;15(3):1939–44.

23. Bray RA. Flow cytometry crossmatching for solid organ transplantation. Methods Cell Biol 1994;41:103–19.

24. Bray RA, Lebeck LK, Gebel HM. The flow cytometric crossmatch. Dual-color analysis of T cell and B cell reactivities. Transplantation 1989;48(5):834–40.

25. Scornik JC, Bray RA, Pollack MS, et al. Multicenter evaluation of the flow cytometry T-cell crossmatch: results from the American Society of Histocompatibility and Immunogenetics-College of American Pathologists proficiency testing program. Transplantation 1997;63(10):1440–5.

26. Lazda VA, Pollak R, Mozes MF, et al. The relationship between flow cytometer crossmatch results and subsequent rejection episodes in cadaver renal allograft recipients. Transplantation 1988;45(3):562–5.

27. Mahoney RJ, Ault KA, Given SR, et al. The flow cytometric crossmatch and early renal transplant loss. Transplantation 1990;49(3):527–35.

28. Talbot D, Givan AL, Shenton BK, et al. The relevance of a more sensitive crossmatch assay to renal transplantation. Transplantation 1989;47(3):552–5.

29. Karpinski M, Rush D, Jeffery J, et al. Flow cytometric crossmatching in primary renal transplant recipients with a negative anti-human globulin enhanced cytotoxicity crossmatch. J Am Soc Nephrol 2001;12(12):2807–14.

30. Bray RA. Flow cytometry in the transplant laboratory. Ann N Y Acad Sci 1993;677: 138–51.

31. Bray RA. Flow cytometry in human leukocyte antigen testing. Semin Hematol 2001;38(2):194–200.

32. Bray RA, Gebel HM, Ellis TM. Flow cytometric assessment of HLA alloantibodies. Curr Protoc Cytom 2004;Chapter 6. Unit 6. 16.

33. Bearden CM, Agarwal A, Book BK, et al. Pronase treatment facilitates alloanti-body flow cytometric and cytotoxic crossmatching in the presence of rituximab. Hum Immunol 2004;65(8):803–9.
34. Desoutter J, Apithy MJ, Bartczak S, et al. False positive B-cells crossmatch after prior rituximab exposure of the kidney donor. Case Rep Transplant 2016;2016: 4534898.
35. Desoutter J, Apithy MJ, Guillaume N. Unexpected positive prospective cross-matches in organ transplant. Exp Clin Transplant 2017;15(3):253–9.
36. Szewczyk K, Barrios K, Magas D, et al. Flow cytometry crossmatch reactivity with pronase-treated T cells induced by non-HLA autoantibodies in human immunode-ficiency virus-infected patients. Hum Immunol 2016;77(6):449–55.
37. Apps R, Meng Z, Del Prete GQ, et al. Relative expression levels of the HLA class-I proteins in normal and HIV-infected cells. J Immunol 2015;194(8):3594–600.
38. Ciurea SO, Thall PF, Wang X, et al. Donor-specific anti-HLA Abs and graft failure in matched unrelated donor hematopoietic stem cell transplantation. Blood 2011; 118(22):5957–64.
39. Pellegrino MA, Belvedere M, Pellegrino AG, et al. B peripheral lymphocytes ex-press more HLA antigens than T peripheral lymphocytes. Transplantation 1978; 25(2):93–5.
40. Yarzabek B, Zaitouna AJ, Olson E, et al. Variations in HLA-B cell surface expres-sion, half-life and extracellular antigen receptivity. eLife 2018;7:e34961.
41. Petersdorf EW, Gooley TA, Malkki M, et al. HLA-C expression levels define permissible mismatches in hematopoietic cell transplantation. Blood 2014; 124(26):3996–4003.
42. Montagner J, Tarasconi H, Wurdig J, et al. The positive virtual crossmatch. Cor-relation between HLA DSA and flow cytometry crossmatch results. Hum Immunol 2016;77(Suppl):6.
43. Cresswell P. Regulation of HLA class I and class II antigen expression. Br Med Bull 1987;43(1):66–80.
44. Kao KJ, Riley WJ. Genetic predetermination of quantitative expression of HLA an-tigens in platelets and mononuclear leukocytes. Hum Immunol 1993;38(4): 243–50.
45. Vandiedonck C, Taylor MS, Lockstone HE, et al. Pervasive haplotypic variation in the spliceo-transcriptome of the human major histocompatibility complex. Genome Res 2011;21(7):1042–54.
46. Good DJ, Zhang A, Kemesky J, et al. Previously believed to be nonsensical crossmatch results, explained by anti-HLA-C antibodies. Hum Immunol 2017; 78(Suppl):75.
47. Lucas DP, Vega RM, Jackson AM. Variable expression of HLA-C impacts T versus B cell crossmatch outcomes. Hum Immunol 2016;77(Suppl):2.
48. Badders JL, Jones JA, Jeresano ME, et al. Variable HLA expression on deceased donor lymphocytes: not all crossmatches are created equal. Hum Immunol 2015; 76(11):795–800.
49. Basham TY, Merigan TC. Recombinant interferon-gamma increases HLA-DR syn-thesis and expression. J Immunol 1983;130(4):1492–4.
50. Kuipers HF, Biesta PJ, Groothuis TA, et al. Statins affect cell-surface expression of major histocompatibility complex class II molecules by disrupting cholesterol-containing microdomains. Hum Immunol 2005;66(6):653–65.
51. Le Morvan C, Cogne M, Troutaud D, et al. Modification of HLA expression on pe-ripheral lymphocytes and monocytes during aging. Mech Ageing Dev 1998; 105(3):209–20.

52. Viallard JF, Bloch-Michel C, Neau-Cransac M, et al. HLA-DR expression on lymphocyte subsets as a marker of disease activity in patients with systemic lupus erythematosus. Clin Exp Immunol 2001;125(3):485–91.
53. Liwski RS, Greenshields AL, Conrad DM, et al. Rapid optimized flow cytometric crossmatch (FCXM) assays: the halifax and halifaster protocols. Hum Immunol 2018;79(1):28–38.
54. Barrios K, Lunz J, Labuda B, et al. Optimized flow cytometry crossmatch with increased sensitivity and specificity. Am J Transplant 2016;16(Suppl):609.
55. Lobo PI, Spencer CE, Stevenson WC, et al. The use of pronase-digested human leukocytes to improve specificity of the flow cytometric crossmatch. Transpl Int 1995;8(6):472–80.
56. Vaidya S, Cooper TY, Avandsalehi J, et al. Improved flow cytometric detection of HLA alloantibodies using pronase: potential implications in renal transplantation. Transplantation 2001;71(3):422–8.
57. Hetrick SJ, Schillinger KP, Zachary AA, et al. Impact of pronase on flow cytometric crossmatch outcome. Hum Immunol 2011;72(4):330–6.
58. Park H, Lim YM, Han BY, et al. Frequent false-positive reactions in pronase-treated T-cell flow cytometric cross-match tests. Transplant Proc 2012;44(1):87–90.
59. Hardt M, Baron T, Groschup MH. A comparative study of immunohistochemical methods for detecting abnormal prion protein with monoclonal and polyclonal antibodies. J Comp Pathol 2000;122(1):43–53.
60. Lipman NS, Jackson LR, Trudel LJ, et al. Monoclonal versus polyclonal antibodies: distinguishing characteristics, applications, and information resources. ILAR J 2005;46(3):258–68.
61. Kerman RH, Van Buren CT, Lewis RM, et al. Improved graft survival for flow cytometry and antihuman globulin crossmatch-negative retransplant recipients. Transplantation 1990;49(1):52–6.

Human Leukocyte Antigen Epitope Matching in Solid Organ Transplantation

Matthew F. Cusick, PhD, D(ABHI)[a],*, Peter T. Jindra, PhD, D(ABHI)[b]

KEYWORDS

• Epitope • T cell • B cell • Allorecognition • Transplantation

KEY POINTS

• HLA epitope matching is a marked upgrade over counting HLA mismatches.
• Vaccinology computer programs can be used to study immunogenicity and these findings correlate with a characterized HLA epitope.
• More structural data are needed to train these computer algorithms, which may increase the predictive value.
• Mechanistic studies should be performed to prove theoretic epitopes.
• There are acknowledged limitations to these predictive computer algorithms and more information is clearly needed to ensure these approaches are equitable and safe to use in clinical diagnostics.

INTRODUCTION

Recent attempts are being made in the transplant community to develop computational methods using epitope matching to determine donor-recipient compatibility in solid organ transplantation. The alloimmune response is multifactorial, involving host immune response genes, cellular responses (eg, monocytes, natural killer cells, T cells), humoral responses (B cells), cytokines, and other factors (eg, viral infections, ethnicity). Most of these computer algorithms are attempting to incorporate these complex and interrelated responses into a quantifiable number to determine risk and compatibility.

The most recognized genes to be involved in an alloimmune response are the human leukocyte antigen (HLA) genes located on chromosome 6. These genes encode for major histocompatibility complex (MHC) molecules that are expressed on the cell surface and coordinate the adaptive immune system, which protects against foreign

Disclosure: The authors have nothing to disclose.
[a] Immune Evaluation Laboratory, Baylor College of Medicine, One Baylor Plaza, MS:BCM 504, Houston, TX 77030, USA; [b] Department of Surgery, Immune Evaluation Laboratory, Baylor College of Medicine, One Baylor Plaza, MS:BCM 504, Houston, TX 77030, USA
* Corresponding author.
E-mail address: Matthew.Cusick@bcm.edu

microbes, or non-self. There are 2 classic HLA antigens, class I and class II. The HLA class I and II molecules, expressed on the surface of antigen-presenting cells, present peptide to a T-cell receptor (TCR) on $CD8^+$ or $CD4^+$ T cells, respectively. The engagement of the TCR by the peptide-MHC complex is necessary for the activation of $CD4^+$ and $CD8^+$ T cells, thereby leading to an effective cellular immune response, which includes the subsequent activation of B cells. B cells that specifically bind native protein antigens differentiate into plasma cells that secrete high amounts of antibody directed against the immunizing antigen. In transplantation, recent advances in cell-depleting pharmacologic agents has lessened the effect of T cells in acute rejection; however, it is clear that donor-specific antibodies (DSAs) produced by B/plasma cells are deleterious to allograft survival, both in the short-term and long-term, with no effective treatment modalities to eliminate memory B-cell and plasma-cell responses.[1–5]

Immunologic assessment, determining donor-recipient compatibility, involves multiple HLA techniques for assessing the risk of rejection against a specific donor. The current practice used by most centers relies on both characterization of anti-HLA antibodies in a patient's serum, using in vitro bead-based assays, and molecular typing of donor HLA antigens, to determine if a patient has antibodies to a specific donor's HLA. Historically, both patient and donor HLA typing and characterization of anti-HLA antibodies in a patient's serum was done serologically using appropriate antisera and well-characterized cell types. However, recent advances in molecular typing and antibody detection have increased our knowledge of the HLA system and a patient's sensitization status. Currently, the approach to determine "HLA match grade" is to count the number of HLA-A, HLA-B, and HLA-DR mismatches between a donor and recipient. This is a very narrow approach that does not account for mismatches at HLA-C, HLA-DQA/DQB, HLA-DPA, or HLA-DPB nor allele-specific differences within each HLA loci. Recently, there has been a movement in the field of transplantation toward using HLA epitope matching to assess immunologic risk, "HLA match grade," and to direct the allocation of organs. This approach, similar to counting HLA mismatches, has focused primarily on quantifying the number of potential epitope mismatches and subsequently correlating this number of epitope mismatches to the development of de novo DSAs (dnDSA) and allograph survival.

Fusion of the knowledge gained on the molecular level with what has been characterized serologically has been pushing the field toward using "epitope-matching" programs and, even if these approaches are not fully accepted, these computer programs are being used to determine alloimmune risk in clinical diagnostics. There are several recent reviews[6–9] that provide excellent insight into the available programs that can be used for HLA matching. Therefore, in this review, we discuss recent advances in HLA "matching" and expand on some of the immunologic challenges limiting the efficacy of these epitope-matching programs.

ANTIBODY STRUCTURE AND FUNCTION

B-cell receptors (BCRs) are immunoglobulins (Ig) presented on the surface of B cells that are responsible for specific antigen recognition and binding. The receptors are composed of 2 identical heavy (H) polypeptide chains ($\sim$500 amino acid residues) covalently linked by disulfide bonds to the light (L) polypeptide chains ($\sim$250 amino acid residues). Both the H and L chains have a variable (V) region at the N-terminal portion and a constant (C) region at the C-terminal portion (**Fig. 1**). The H chain has 4 to 5 domains (V_H, C_H1, C_H2, C_H3, C_H4) depending on the isotype, in that IgM and IgE each contain a C_H4 domain, and the L chain is made up of 2 domains (V_L and C_L). The H chain has 5 isotypes defined by the structural differences at the C region

(IgG, IgA, IgM, IgE, and IgD; the latter 2 of which are minimally present in normal serum). The L chain domains are disulfide-linked to the V_H and C_H1 to form the Fab (fragment antigen-binding) region and linked to the Fc (fragment crystallizable) region via noncovalent association of the C_H2-3/4 regions from both H chains.

The V region of each H and L chain contains 3 hypervariable sequences: the complementarity-determining regions (CDRs). Antibody recognition specificity is the result of the 3-dimensional (3D) structures formed by these 6 CDRs (3 from each H and L chain), termed paratopes or antigen-binding sites, being able to specifically bind to complementary regions (epitopes) on antigens. Although the Fabs have a limited number of canonical structures, the usage of CDRs increases the variability in antigen-antibody specificity. The surface area of the V region is approximately 280 nm^2 ($\sim$50–70 amino acid residues) compared with 30 to 110 nm^2 ($\sim$15–20 amino acid residues) for a paratope (antigen-binding site). This indicates that an antibody may contain several paratopes capable of binding to different epitopes either on the same antigen or another antigen, but in certain instances steric hindrance could prevent an antibody simultaneously binding to 2 antigen molecules at the same time. However, if 2 paratope subsites do not overlap, an antibody molecule could potentially bind simultaneously to 2 small antigens.[10] Taking this into consideration, antibodies are most likely not monospecific. Antigen-antibody binding leads to activation of signaling cascades within the target cells, activation of the complement cascade, and attachment of antibody to immune cells through Fc receptors. Varying degrees of functionality are dependent on the affinity and avidity of the antibody.

WHAT IS AN EPITOPE?

The adaptive immune response to a foreign microbe involves both B cells recognizing native protein antigens and differentiating into antibody-producing plasma cells and T cells binding to unfolded peptide fragments derived from the processing of antigen within antigen-presenting cells. TCRs specifically bind to these peptide fragments when presented in the groove of MHC.

The primary antibody repertoire mainly consists of IgM molecules before exogenous antigen exposure. On exposure to a foreign antigen, B cells recognize antigens via their membrane-bound Ig receptors (BCRs), leading to the production of antigen-specific antibodies. Therefore, an antigen is any molecule that is bound by a BCR or an antibody molecule and the antigen residue bound by the antibody is called a B-cell epitope or antigenic determinant. Protein antigen epitopes may be either continuous: a short peptide from the protein sequence (linear), or discontinuous: a

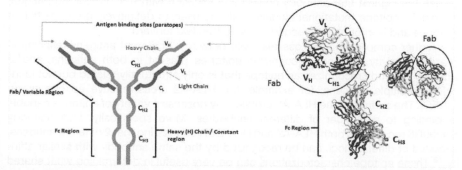

Fig. 1. Schematic (*left*) and crystal structure (*right*) of an intact monoclonal mouse antibody (PDB ID: 1IGT).

patch of atoms on the protein surface in 3D space (conformational). Crystallographic studies of antibody-protein complexes have shown that most epitopes are discontinuous. Confounding the issue of defining an epitope is that there are protein post-translational modifications and nonprotein epitopes, such as polysaccharides, DNA, glycoproteins, and other molecules, which, to date, have not been incorporated into any algorithms. However, for this review, we focused primarily on protein-protein interactions.

ANTIBODY SPECIFICITY: A BIASED CHARACTERIZATION

The specificity of antigen-antibody recognition has evolved from an all-or-nothing model to a goodness-of-fit between molecules having varying degrees of stereochemical complementarity.[11,12] Specificity is determined by an antibody's ability to discriminate between different antigens.[13] Therefore, an antibody's specificity is dependent on what a researcher chooses to compare a particular antibody's response against; this comparison should be acknowledged as a biased approach. The most accepted approach for identifying epitopes and paratopes is through determination of the 3D structure of antigen-antibody complexes, allowing for a more accurate identification of B-cell epitopes; however, this is currently not a feasible approach for every potential interaction due to time and technical constraints. Therefore, the current practice for identification of anti-HLA antibodies in patient sera is through the use of synthetic beads coated with HLA antigens: single-antigen beads (SABs). The specificity is determined by comparing that reactivity against the other antigen-coated beads on a particular panel.

Briefly, the output of SABs is mean fluorescence intensity (MFI), and there is no consensus as to what is considered "positive" between centers.[2,14] It has been proposed that titrating serum to determine antibody strength is an approach for measuring antibody strength over time, monitoring antibody levels pre-desensitization and post-desensitization, and for predicting treatment outcome.[15,16] However, this approach, as with using the raw MFI value, is still denoting strength using the MFI. This complicates the use of certain algorithms due to certain programs incorporating these MFI results into what could be an acceptable mismatch without a functional cell-based assay.

Using the premise that an antibody is never specific for the entire HLA antigen as a whole, but for an epitope, it has been presumed that the stimulating antigen will induce a higher antibody titer.[17] We propose that the information obtained from dilution studies may provide valuable insight into the specificity and selectivity of an antibody, in that, the highest titer antibody could be associated with the immunizing antigen. Ultimately, epitope mutational studies could be used to definitively prove particular epitopes and is information needed to move the field forward.

A further complication is cross-reactivity between 2 different antigens resulting in shared reactivity, antibody recognizing epitopes present in both antigens, and/or when an antibody recognizes an epitope that is only structurally related but not identical in multiple antigens; for example, the HLA-A2 cross-reactive epitope group (CREG). The surface of the HLA-A2 protein may possess a variety of epitopes capable of binding to a number of different antibodies. More specifically, HLA antibody SN230G6 recognizes both HLA-A2 and HLA-B57, suggesting that 2 different antigens, encoded at different loci, can be recognized by the same antibody with similar affinity.[18] These epitope characterizations can be very useful in determining what shared epitopes are to be avoided, but patients demonstrating some partial reactivity, such as the HLA-A68 private epitope, which is not shared with CREG member HLA-A2, may potentially deny a patient an organ due the lack of information on the physiologic relevance of only partially shared epitope(s). However, IgG antibodies can be highly specific for an antigen and in certain cases, in which there is a single amino acid substitution, can lead to the antibody not being able to recognize the mutated antigen. On the other hand, anti-HLA IgG antibodies can be cross-reactive with a similar antigen, which complicates the interpretation of results derived in an HLA laboratory.

Another issue associated with using the numerical approach of epitope counting is epitope spreading. As discussed previously, B cells bind to specific epitopes through the BCR and protein, and protein complexes can be internalized. These internalized proteins, potentially containing other epitopes in addition to the epitope(s) recognized by the BCR, are processed, and subsequently these peptides are bound to MHC class II molecules and presented at the surface of the cell. This can induce a variety of different T-cell and B-cell specificities that effectively direct (or spread) the immune response against other parts of the antigen, even against nonaccessible parts of the antigen. This is one mechanism that has been shown to be involved in breaking tolerance to self, such as is seen in type 1 diabetes and multiple sclerosis.[19,20] Anecdotal evidence on non-HLA antibodies causing damage to allografts suggests that alloimmune responses work synergistically with tissue-specific responses to promote graft rejection. This may occur by alloreactive CD8[+] T cells and alloantibodies causing tissue damage, which may cause the release of sequestered self-tissue antigens. Subsequently, these peptides could be processed via the MHC class II pathway, inducing a cellular and humoral response. Although there are a number of potential autoimmune antigens implicated, for example, Vimentin,[21] further investigation is needed to determine if these antibodies are associated with an autoimmune and/or alloimmune response or if these are the result of a previous infectious agent inducing a cross-reactive response with a host cell determinant, termed molecular mimicry.[22,23] Regardless, the detection of these antibodies and characterization of these epitopes has not been incorporated into epitope matching.

B-CELL EPITOPE PREDICTION ISSUES: IMMUNOGENIC EPITOPES?

Although higher resolution sequencing of HLA loci is becoming a reality, this approach will not resolve certain issues associated with identifying epitopes, mainly because these methods have limited information to predict discontinuous epitopes. As stated previously, most B-cell epitopes are 3D and the prediction of these types of epitopes is mainly dependent on the protein 3D structure of antigen-antibody complexes. Paradoxically, next-generation sequencing of the HLA loci, which provides the "linear" or sequence results, is a major technological advancement in clinical diagnostics, while not providing any relevant data on antibody responsiveness that was provided by serologic typing. Furthermore, a significant drawback to this approach is that very few well-characterized antigen-antibody structures are available; thereby limiting the efficacy of these approaches. However, the information gained from other 3D crystallography studies, not related to alloantibody-HLA antigen, has been incorporated into certain B-cell epitope prediction models. These approaches may offer insight into predicting potential B-cell epitopes in silico.

It has been postulated that permissible HLA mismatches are due to a lower antigenic load between donor/recipient pairs.[3,24] The premise is based on different HLAs sharing individual epitopes that will not induce an alloimmune response, compared with mismatched epitopes driving an alloimmune response. Therefore, quantifying the number of epitope mismatches between donor and recipient is potentially a better method to determine HLA match grade compared with counting the number of HLA mismatches to predict alloimmune risk.[3,25–27] There are several available HLA programs, including HLAMatchmaker and PIRCHE-II (HLA class II–restricted predicted recognizable HLA epitopes). The basic premise of these computer algorithms is that there will be no alloimmune response to self-HLA antigens.

For antibody epitopes, Rene Duquesnoy[28–30] developed the most widely used computer algorithm, HLAMatchmaker. The premise of this program is that a cluster of polymorphic (non-self) amino acids within a 3.0 to 3.5-Å radius of an antibody-accessible sequence position, termed an eplet, may induce an antibody response. Eplets are defined as small patches of amino acids exposed on the surface of an HLA antigen that are hypothesized to be important for antigen/antibody binding. The algorithm subtracts self-HLA eplets based on the assumption that antibodies cannot be made against self. This program quantifies the number of eplet mismatches associated with mismatched donor HLA antigen and allows for potential alloimmune response risk associated with this eplet mismatch number.

Currently, the focus is on determining the binding capacity of an epitope or antigen, which is based on chemical interactions (ie, epitope-paratope recognition). Using available information obtained from SAB results and determining patient reactivity to particular HLAs has led to the extrapolation of the immunogenicity based on the number of HLA eplet mismatches. This is most likely a distortion of the biological process dictated by the immune response to a particular antigen and is also likely an independent process from antigenicity. Therefore, multiple parameters should be considered when assessing if a particular antigen may be immunogenic. In addition, antigenicity (ability to bind) and immunogenicity (ability to induce a response) are not always directly associated with the exact same region on a protein molecule. The current tools allow us to assess eplet load between donor and recipients while making the assumption that a higher eplet burden leads to a higher risk of developing a de novo anti-HLA antibody. Future test development is needed to determine which epitope mismatches are most immunogenic so we can pinpoint which eplets need to be avoided, instead of the overall number of eplet differences. Importantly, more studies examining eplet diversity in more diverse populations are needed to equitably determine eplet mismatches and immunogenicity.

Recent data suggest that the configuration of amino acids in an epitope/eplet, even when the amino acids are shared between donor and recipient, may have an effect on inducing an immune response and antibody binding.[31–33] Interestingly, Kosmoliaptsis and colleagues[34–36] have shown that both the number of eplet mismatches and the number of polymorphic amino acid mismatches were predictors of dnDSA. Furthermore, this group has demonstrated that certain amino acid characteristics, such as hydrophobicity and electrostatic charge of the side chains, are important factors in predicting immunogenicity. They have developed both the hydrophobicity match score and electrostatic mismatch score. Their results appear to be strong predictors for the development of dnDSA formation in renal transplant recipients, suggesting this approach could be a superior predictor of dnDSA compared with eplet mismatches and amino acid mismatches; however, these results require further investigation.[34–36]

B-CELL AND T-CELL AXIS

The humoral response is directly responsible for chronic rejection through the formation of DSA. In addition, allospecific B cells may have an indirect role in chronic rejection. These B cells may have a heightened capacity to capture and process allo-antigens. These alloantigens are shed from the graft, processed, and presented as peptides in the context of self-MHC class II molecules (indirect allorecognition) at the cell surface. Activated CD4$^+$ T cells, recognizing a specific alloantigen-MHC mole-cule, provide the necessary help, signals, and cytokines, to the B cells to proliferate and differentiate into anti-HLA IgG-producing plasma cells. The PIRCHE-II computa-tional algorithm indirectly predicts recognizable HLA-derived donor peptides that may induce the production of DSA. The efficacy of this program has been described in renal transplant recipients in whom a correlation was shown between a low PIRCHE-II number and low detection of DSA.[37] However, this program, although showing tremendous promise as a predictive tool on the population level, has not translated over to clinical relevance for individual patients because of no high-resolution HLA typing; HLA-DRB3/4/5, HLA-DQA/DQB, and HLA-DPA/DPB were not incorporated into the algorithm; a low PIRCHE-II score did not necessarily mean freedom from developing dnDSA, whereas conversely a high PIRCHE-II was not a definitive risk factor for the development of dnDSA; and there was no consideration of splice variants of HLA. Taken together, using these programs in combination may be the best approach to determine antigenicity and immunogenicity, but the real ques-tion is how to use these results in clinical diagnostics in an equitable and sage manner.

APPLYING VACCINOLOGY TO TRANSPLANT IMMUNOLOGY

Tremendous effort has been put toward T-cell and B-cell epitope discovery for vac-cine design. Clearly, the programs discussed previously are similar to other bioinfor-matics tools associated with epitope discovery and vaccine design. As with the HLA epitope programs, the Immune Epitope Database and Analysis Resource is freely available to all researchers and has numerous applications for epitope analysis and prediction tools; please refer to Flerl and colleagues[38] for a more comprehensive re-view. There are prediction tools used to predict MHC class I and II immunogenicity and for predicting linear and discontinuous B-cell epitopes. At first glance, vaccine design and transplantation do not appear to be related; however, the immunologic "goals" are the same: to characterize or predict if memory T-cell and B-cell responses are induced to a particular antigen. For vaccine design, the goal is to determine how to induce memory against a foreign antigen. Conversely, transplantation is trying to determine how to prevent a memory response against an antigen. Therefore, the goal in transplantation is to have an anti-vaccine that will induce tolerance to a graft. So, can we exploit what we know about vaccines and apply this to alloimmunity?

There are several B-cell epitope prediction tools that we evaluate in relation to pre-viously characterized HLA epitopes. BepiPred is a machine-learning algorithm designed to predict linear B-cell epitopes.[39] Certain physicochemical amino acid properties incorporated into determining B-cell epitopes are hydrophobicity,[40] surface accessibility,[41] beta-turns,[42] and flexibility (reviewed in Ref.[38]). DiscoTope 2.0 is a computer-based algorithm, one of many, used to determine discontinuous B-cell epi-topes.[43,44] DiscoTope 2.0 is designed to use the protein's geometric properties and is programmed using numerous X-ray crystal structures of antibody-protein complexes. It assigns every residue a score using multiple parameters, including normalized values from Parker's hydrophilicity scale, amino acid propensity, number of contacts within 10 Å, and relative solvent accessibility. In addition, the program needs the Pro-tein Data Bank (PDB) identification (ID), the crystal structure of interest, to use the pro-gram. If there is no 3D structure available in the PDB, there are homology modeling programs available to build theoretic crystal structures of antigens and antibodies.

To explore if these 2 programs were able to identify similar regions of an HLA antigen associated with characterized HLA epitopes, we used HLA-DQ8 structure and input this into DiscoTope 2.0 and BepiPred. Overall, the characterized DQ8β epitopes listed in the HLA epitope registry (http://www.epregistry.com.br/) were identified as immunogenic with either the DiscoTope 2.0 (discontinuous) or BepiPred (linear) programs (**Fig. 2**). These programs have a number of issues, in that they are not designed to subtract potential self-epitopes, thereby resulting in a marked increase in potential B-cell epitopes. Furthermore, both BepiPred and DiscoTope 2.0 have been shown to have relatively poor prediction performance, potentially due to the limited number of 3D structures available to "train" the algorithms. It should be noted that, to our knowledge, there are no crystal structures of an alloantibody binding to an HLA molecule. Taken together, these tools are important in advancing our knowledge, but the predictive performance is limited by the lack of 3D structure information, raising this very important question: how predictive are the HLA-matching epitope programs?

IS HLA MATCHING JUST A NUMBERS GAME?

Due to advances in immunosuppression, there was a paradigm shift from matching at donor-recipient HLA loci to detecting the presence of donor-specific anti-HLA antibodies. Focusing on long-term graft outcomes, the field appears to be circling back to the idea that HLA matching, even in the presence of immunosuppression, has a long-term benefit. Lower eplet mismatch loads in DR and DQ lead to less de novo anti-HLA antibody production and extended graft survival.[27] However, the available prediction tools are limited, mainly due to the lack of relevant information to "train" these computer algorithms; that is, crystal structures. The immune response to a graft is a dynamic process consisting of the innate and adaptive immune response. The detection of antibodies against an antigen is the end product of this complex process. Although these epitope-matching programs appear to be a significant improvement in determining immunologic risk and compatibility, it is currently unclear whether fewer eplet mismatches is the most appropriate approach toward determining immunogenicity. Other very significant issues needing to be addressed are (1) how would this approach impact recipient wait times, (2) would this limit access to minority populations because they inherently have increased eplet mismatches to the

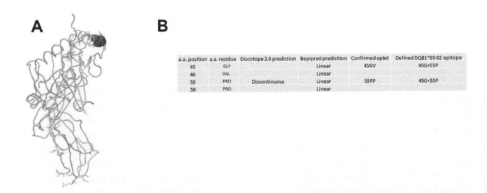

A   **B**

a.a. position	a.a. residue	Discotope 2.0 prediction	Bepipred prediction	Confirmed eplet	Defined DQB1*03:02 epitope
45	GLY		Linear	45GV	45G+55P
46	VAL		Linear		
55	PRO	Discontinuous	Linear	55PP	45G+55P
56	PRO		Linear		

Fig. 2. Representative example of predicted B-cell epitopes using both linear and discontinuous computer programs. (*A*) Crystal structure of DQ8 (PBD ID: 1JK8). The red area is the 45GV eplet. (*B*) Representative example of the prediction results of DiscoTope 2.0, BepiPred, and confirmed eplets found on http://www.epregistry.com/br.

predominately White donor pool, and (3) does epitope matching provide more permissible HLA antigen mismatches compared with current HLA-matching practices?

SUMMARY

The detection of an anti-HLA antibody against a particular antigen does not necessarily relate to the immunogenic capacity of a particular antigen to induce the same antibody in another person. Therein lies a fundamental problem with the current approach in HLA epitope matching, in that the detection of HLA antibodies or differences in HLA does not tell you what particular non–self-component of an antigen is capable of inducing an immune response in another person, which is the end goal. This is especially true in patients with antibody reactivity to numerous HLA antigens, such as women and minorities. Overall, HLA epitope matching is being incorporated as a tool for assessing immunologic risk and as an adjuvant when certain alleles are not represented on the SAB panels. Clearly, more information is needed to continue this rapid advancement in HLA epitope matching, including more 3D structural data and mechanistic studies characterizing HLA epitopes.

ACKNOWLEDGMENTS

The authors thank Jane E. Libbey, MS, for copyediting and proofreading the article.

REFERENCES

1. Terasaki PI, Ozawa M. Predicting kidney graft failure by HLA antibodies: a prospective trial. Am J Transplant 2004;4(3):438–43.
2. Tait BD, Susal C, Gebel HM, et al. Consensus guidelines on the testing and clinical management issues associated with HLA and non-HLA antibodies in transplantation. Transplantation 2013;95(1):19–47.
3. Wiebe C, Nickerson P. Posttransplant monitoring of de novo human leukocyte antigen donor-specific antibodies in kidney transplantation. Curr Opin Organ Transplant 2013;18(4):470–7.
4. Everly MJ, Rebellato LM, Haisch CE, et al. Incidence and impact of de novo donor-specific alloantibody in primary renal allografts. Transplantation 2013; 95(3):410–7.
5. Terasaki PI. A personal perspective: 100-year history of the humoral theory of transplantation. Transplantation 2012;93(8):751–6.
6. Kramer CSM, Roelen DL, Heidt S, et al. Defining the immunogenicity and antigenicity of HLA epitopes is crucial for optimal epitope matching in clinical renal transplantation. HLA 2017;90(1):5–16.
7. Sypek M, Kausman J, Holt S, et al. HLA epitope matching in kidney transplantation: an overview for the general nephrologist. Am J Kidney Dis 2017;17:31016–8.
8. El-Awar N, Jucaud V, Nguyen A. HLA epitopes: the targets of monoclonal and alloantibodies defined. J Immunol Res 2017;2017:3406230.
9. Lim WH, Wong G, Heidt S, et al. Novel aspects of epitope matching and practical application in kidney transplantation. Kidney Int 2018;93(2):314–24.
10. Bhattacharjee AK, Glaudemans CP. Dual binding specificities in MOPC 384 and 870 murine myeloma immunoglobulins. J Immunol 1978;120(2):411–3.
11. Silverstein AM. History of immunology: development of the concept of immunologic specificity: II. Cell Immunol 1982;71(1):183–95.
12. Silverstein AM. History of immunology. Development of the concept of immunologic specificity, I. Cell Immunol 1982;67(2):396–409.

13. Van Regenmortel MH. Specificity, polyspecificity, and heterospecificity of antibody-antigen recognition. J Mol Recognit 2014;27(11):627–39.
14. Reed EF, Rao P, Zhang Z, et al. Comprehensive assessment and standardization of solid phase multiplex-bead arrays for the detection of antibodies to HLA. Am J Transplant 2013;13(7):1859–70.
15. Tambur AR, Herrera ND, Haarberg KM, et al. Assessing antibody strength: comparison of MFI, C1q, and titer information. Am J Transplant 2015;15(9):2421–30.
16. Walsh RC, Brailey P, Girnita A, et al. Early and late acute antibody-mediated rejection differ immunologically and in response to proteasome inhibition. Transplantation 2011;91(11):1218–26.
17. Richards FF, Konigsberg WH, Rosenstein RW, et al. On the specificity of antibodies. Science 1975;187(4172):130–7.
18. Daga S, Moyse H, Briggs D, et al. Direct quantitative measurement of the kinetics of HLA-specific antibody interactions with isolated HLA proteins. Hum Immunol 2017;79(2):122–8.
19. McRae BL, Vanderlugt CL, Dal Canto MC, et al. Functional evidence for epitope spreading in the relapsing pathology of experimental autoimmune encephalomyelitis. J Exp Med 1995;182(1):75–85.
20. Tisch R, Yang XD, Singer SM, et al. Immune response to glutamic acid decarboxylase correlates with insulitis in non-obese diabetic mice. Nature 1993;366(6450): 72–5.
21. Jurcevic S, Ainsworth ME, Pomerance A, et al. Antivimentin antibodies are an independent predictor of transplant-associated coronary artery disease after cardiac transplantation. Transplantation 2001;71(7):886–92.
22. Fujinami RS, Oldstone MB, Wroblewska Z, et al. Molecular mimicry in virus infection: crossreaction of measles virus phosphoprotein or of herpes simplex virus protein with human intermediate filaments. Proc Natl Acad Sci U S A 1983; 80(8):2346–50.
23. Cusick MF, Libbey JE, Fujinami RS. Molecular mimicry as a mechanism of autoimmune disease. Clin Rev Allergy Immunol 2012;42(1):102–11.
24. Duquesnoy RJ. HLA epitope based matching for transplantation. Transpl Immunol 2014;31(1):1–6.
25. Bryan CF, Chadha V, Warady BA. Donor selection in pediatric kidney transplantation using DR and DQ eplet mismatching: a new histocompatibility paradigm. Pediatr Transplant 2016;20(7):926–30.
26. Kausman JY, Walker AM, Cantwell LS, et al. Application of an epitope-based allocation system in pediatric kidney transplantation. Pediatr Transplant 2016;20(7): 931–8.
27. Wiebe C, Pochinco D, Blydt-Hansen TD, et al. Class II HLA epitope matching—a strategy to minimize de novo donor-specific antibody development and improve outcomes. Am J Transplant 2013;13(12):3114–22.
28. Duquesnoy RJ. A structurally based approach to determine HLA compatibility at the humoral immune level. Hum Immunol 2006;67(11):847–62.
29. Duquesnoy RJ, Askar M. HLAMatchmaker: a molecularly based algorithm for histocompatibility determination. V. Eplet matching for HLA-DR, HLA-DQ, and HLA-DP. Hum Immunol 2007;68(1):12–25.
30. Duquesnoy RJ. HLAMMATCHMAKER: a molecularly based donor selection algorithm for highly alloimmunized patients. Transplant Proc 2001;33(1–2):493–7.
31. El-Awar N, Terasaki PI, Cai J, et al. Epitopes of HLA-A, B, C, DR, DQ, DP and MICA antigens. Clin Transpl 2009;295–321.

32. Duquesnoy RJ, Marrari M, Mulder A, et al. First report on the antibody verification of HLA-ABC epitopes recorded in the website-based HLA epitope registry. Tissue Antigens 2014;83(6):391–400.
33. Duquesnoy RJ, Marrari M, Tambur AR, et al. First report on the antibody verification of HLA-DR, HLA-DQ and HLA-DP epitopes recorded in the HLA epitope registry. Hum Immunol 2014;75(11):1097–103.
34. Kosmoliaptsis V, Chaudhry AN, Sharples LD, et al. Predicting HLA class I alloantigen immunogenicity from the number and physiochemical properties of amino acid polymorphisms. Transplantation 2009;88(6):791–8.
35. Kosmoliaptsis V, Mallon DH, Chen Y, et al. Alloantibody responses after renal transplant failure can be better predicted by donor-recipient HLA amino acid sequence and physicochemical disparities than conventional HLA matching. Am J Transplant 2016;16(7):2139–47.
36. Kosmoliaptsis V, Sharples LD, Chaudhry AN, et al. Predicting HLA class II alloantigen immunogenicity from the number and physiochemical properties of amino acid polymorphisms. Transplantation 2011;91(2):183–90.
37. Otten HG, Calis JJ, Kesmir C, et al. Predicted indirectly recognizable HLA epitopes presented by HLA-DR correlate with the de novo development of donor-specific HLA IgG antibodies after kidney transplantation. Hum Immunol 2013; 74(3):290–6.
38. Fleri W, Paul S, Dhanda SK, et al. The immune epitope database and analysis resource in epitope discovery and synthetic vaccine design. Front Immunol 2017;8:278.
39. Larsen JE, Lund O, Nielsen M. Improved method for predicting linear B-cell epitopes. Immunome Res 2006;2:2.
40. Parker JM, Guo D, Hodges RS. New hydrophilicity scale derived from high-performance liquid chromatography peptide retention data: correlation of predicted surface residues with antigenicity and X-ray-derived accessible sites. Biochemistry 1986;25(19):5425–32.
41. Emini EA, Hughes JV, Perlow DS, et al. Induction of hepatitis A virus-neutralizing antibody by a virus-specific synthetic peptide. J Virol 1985;55(3):836–9.
42. Pellequer JL, Van Regenmortel MH. Measurement of kinetic binding constants of viral antibodies using a new biosensor technology. J Immunol Methods 1993; 166(1):133–43.
43. Haste Andersen P, Nielsen M, Lund O. Prediction of residues in discontinuous B-cell epitopes using protein 3D structures. Protein Sci 2006;15(11):2558–67.
44. Kringelum JV, Lundegaard C, Lund O, et al. Reliable B cell epitope predictions: impacts of method development and improved benchmarking. PLoS Comput Biol 2012;8(12):e1002829.

Maintaining the Health of the Renal Allograft
Laboratory and Histologic Monitoring After Kidney Transplantation

Carrie A. Schinstock, MD[a],*, Manish J. Gandhi, MD[b]

KEYWORDS

- Posttransplant monitoring • De novo donor-specific antibodies • Surveillance biopsy
- Posttransplant GFR • Posttransplant proteinuria

KEY POINTS

- Adequate post–kidney transplant monitoring includes kidney function monitoring, infectious disease surveillance, following immunosuppressant drug levels, testing for adverse effects of medications, and screening for common comorbidities.
- De novo donor-specific antibody is associated with antibody-mediated rejection and is an indicator of inadequate immunosuppression (either intended by the prescribing physician or medication nonadherence by the patient).
- Surveillance renal biopsies and testing for donor-specific antibody have prognostic value, but it remains unclear whether the use of these tests for surveillance purposes only leads to improved allograft survival.

INTRODUCTION

Kidney transplantation provides the ultimate renal replacement therapy to patients with end-stage renal disease. Advances in posttransplant care, including new immunosuppressive medications, have led to excellent short-term renal allograft survival. However, there is a small therapeutic window within which the patient and the clinician must balance the risk of rejection, with side effects, such as infection, malignancy, and toxicity. Additionally, transplant recipients often have multiple comorbidities, and to maintain the ongoing health of the patient and the renal allograft necessitates ongoing monitoring of the kidney function and the patients' immune status. Laboratory testing plays a key role in this ongoing monitoring, which includes relatively simple tests, such

Disclosure Statement: KL2 TR002379 National Center for Advancing Translational Science (NCATS)
[a] Department of Internal Medicine, Division of Nephrology and Hypertension, William J von Liebig Center for Transplantation and Clinical Regeneration, Mayo Clinic, 200 1st Street Southwest, Rochester, MN 55905, USA; [b] Division of Transfusion Medicine, Mayo Clinic, 200 1st Street Southwest, Rochester, MN 55905, USA
* Corresponding author.
E-mail address: Schinstock.carrie@mayo.edu

as serum creatinine, to complex tests, such as solid-phase assays, used to monitor for donor-specific antibody and surveillance allograft biopsies.

Before ordering any laboratory test, certain factors must be considered, including the predictive value, risk, cost, and availability of the testing (**Table 1**). The clinician must also consider whether the test result will actually change clinical management or outcome. This consideration is especially important for conditions that are irreversible and lack effective therapies. In other circumstances, the identified condition is treatable, but the patient may not derive survival or quality-of-life benefit because of underlying comorbidities.

The field of kidney transplantation is relatively small. Most of the guidance for laboratory monitoring is from expert opinion based on small observational studies in heterogeneous patient populations. Very few randomized controlled trials have been performed in the field of transplantation, much less on the subject of laboratory monitoring. For the purpose of this article, we discuss routine surveillance posttransplant laboratory monitoring. We cover the options and role of kidney function monitoring, infectious disease surveillance, testing for adverse effects of medications, and screening for common comorbidities (**Table 2**). The specific laboratory monitoring protocol varies depending on the transplant center and the patients' underlying risk for rejection, adverse effects, or comorbidities. We also discuss more controversial monitoring posttransplant, including donor-specific antibody screening and the role surveillance allograft biopsy.

MONITORING OF KIDNEY FUNCTION, ELECTROLYTES, AND IMMUNOSUPPRESSION
Renal Function

Serial monitoring of kidney function is one of the most basic and widely accepted practices for long-term laboratory monitoring following the kidney transplant. The

Table 1 Important considerations before ordering any test	
What is the test's predictive value?	Some tests have low sensitivity or specificities and do not adequately discriminate between health and disease.
What is the risk of testing for the patient?	The potential complications of a test are important to consider, including the risk of bleeding from a kidney biopsy or kidney injury from contrast exposure.
How expensive is the test?	Today many patients do not have insurance or have high deductibles and copayments. If a patient is given an expensive bill for services without seeing significant clinical benefit, the patient may forego other important testing or therapies in the future. Even if the patient is not directly responsible for the test, it is important for the health care system as a whole to be mindful of the value and cost-effectiveness of testing.
Will the test results actually change management?	The ordering provider must consider how the results will change management. Important questions for the ordering provider to ask include the following: Is there an effective therapy available? Will the patient want or tolerate treatment? More importantly, the provider should consider whether the disease or condition can be identified with history and physical alone.

Table 2
Outline of routine surveillance posttransplant laboratory monitoring

Laboratory Testing	Suggested Testing Intervals
Kidney function	
Creatinine and eGFR[a]	Daily until hospital dismissal 2–3 times/week for postoperative week 1–4 Weekly for postoperative month 2–3 Every other week for postoperative week 4–6 Monthly for postoperative month 7–12 Every 2–3 month, thereafter

24-h creatinine clearance
Iohexol/Iothalamate renal
  clearance
Cystatin C
	Consider testing annually posttransplant and correlate with
	  serum creatinine and eGFR. The choice of test depends on
	  the cost and availability in your region

24-h urine protein[a]
Protein-to-creatinine ratio[a]
Microalbumin/creatinine
  ratio[a]
	At least once in first posttransplant month to establish
	  baseline
	Every 3 month in first year
	Annually thereafter
	KDIGO does not specify the choice of test for proteinuria
	Consider more frequent monitoring of proteinuria when
	  recurrent native disease expected

Electrolyte abnormalities	
Potassium Magnesium Bicarbonate	At same interval as serum creatinine and eGFR

Drug levels
  (immunosuppression)
	Every other day immediately postoperation until target drug
	  levels are achieved
	Whenever there is a drug change
	At time of drug change

Common comorbid conditions and medication side effects	
Lipid panel[b]	At baseline When there is a concern for nonadherence or new reasons for hyperlipidemia

Fasting glucose (FG)[a]
Hemoglobin A1c[a]
Oral glucose tolerance[a]
  testing
	All nondiabetic recipients should have FG weekly
	  for 4 week
	FG, HbA1c, and/or oral glucose tolerance every
	  3 month for first year
	Annually after first year

Calcium[a]
Phosphorus[a]
Parathyroid hormone[a]
Vitamin D[a]
	At least weekly calcium and phosphorus posttransplant until
	  stable
	The frequency of calcium, phosphorus, PTH, and
	  25-OH vitamin D is based on allograft function and
	  metabolic bone disease

Complete blood count[a]	Daily for 7 days or until hospital dismissal 2–3 times/week for week 2–4 Weekly for month 2–3 Monthly for month 4–12 Annually or when medications changed that could cause anemia, neutropenia, or thrombocytopenia
Infectious disease surveillance	
Urinalysis and culture	Screening for asymptomatic bacteriuria limited to first 1–3 month posttransplant At time of unexplained increase in creatinine

(continued on next page)

Table 2 (continued)	
Laboratory Testing	**Suggested Testing Intervals**
CMV blood PCR[c]	Weekly for 3–6 month in patients who received a CMV-positive donor kidney who are not receiving prophylaxis Weekly to monitor response to therapy in patients with infection Regular monitoring for 8–12 week after prophylaxis discontinuation
BK blood PCR[a]	Plasma nucleic acid testing monthly for the first 3–6 month Every 3 month for posttransplant month 6–12 At time of allograft dysfunction
EBV blood PCR[a]	Regularly within the first year posttransplant in EBV-negative recipients of EBV-positive organs

Abbreviations: CMV, cytomegalovirus; EBV, Epstein-Barr virus; eGFR, estimated glomerular filtration rate; KDIGO, Kidney Disease: Improving Global Outcomes; PCR, polymerase chain reaction; PTH, parathyroid hormone.
[a] According to KDIGO guidelines.[15]
[b] According to KDIGO guidelines for lipid management.[12]
[c] According to Infectious Disease Community of Practice recommendations.[20]

goal is to identify allograft dysfunction and assess the risk for graft loss. The serum creatinine and associated estimated glomerular filtration rate (GFR) are inexpensive, readily available, and the results can be obtained quickly, thus enabling easy monitoring that provides information regarding the stability of allograft function. The problem is that changes in serum creatinine and estimated GFR are nonspecific and often do not provide an accurate assessment of glomerular filtration rate in kidney transplant recipients.

To obtain a more accurate assessment of renal function, inulin, iothalamate, or iohexol clearances can be performed. The advantage of improved accuracy for assessing renal function must be balanced with the increased cost, decreased availability, and increased time of testing. Twenty-hour creatinine clearance can also provide a more accurate assessment of kidney function, but it is cumbersome and can provide inaccurate results if the urine is overcollected or undercollected. This test is also less reliable at a reduced level of GFR when the secretion of creatinine increases.

Another laboratory test used increasingly to estimate GFR is cystatin C. This protein is constantly produced in the human body, freely filtered across the glomerulus, and not secreted by the tubules, making it an ideal endogenous biomarker of kidney function. In the transplant population, 2 cystatin C–based GFR estimating equations have been exclusively derived from a kidney transplant population.[1,2] In the general population, several studies have suggested that serum cystatin C correlates better with GFR than serum creatinine.[2–4] Cystatin C has also been shown to be a stronger predictor of the risk of death and cardiovascular mortality in patients with chronic kidney disease than serum creatinine.[5,6] The limitation of this test is that cystatin C can sometimes be unreliable in settings of high cellular turnover, including cancer,[7] uncontrolled thyroid disease,[8] and steroid therapy.[9,10] This test is more expensive than the serum creatinine and not readily available, which limits its broad use in the transplant community.

Proteinuria

Monitoring for proteinuria is another important aspect of post–kidney transplant monitoring. Identifying new or increasing urine protein can be an early or late indicator of renal allograft damage. Serial monitoring of proteinuria is an integral part of screening for native kidney disease recurrence (ie, for primary focal glomerulosclerosis or membrano-proliferative glomerulonephritis). Especially early posttransplant, it can be difficult to determine whether the urine protein identified is coming from the native kidneys or allograft. Urine protein screening methods include the standard urine dipstick, spot urine protein-to-creatinine ratio, and spot urine albumin-to-creatinine ratio. These tests are readily available, relatively inexpensive, and relatively easy to obtain. The urine dipstick is not quantitative and is relatively insensitive to nonalbumin protein. This test is also prone to false-positive results in the setting of hematuria, antiseptics, recent use of iodinated contrast agents, and high alkaline urine. Because of the limitations of the urine dipstick, spot urine protein and albumin tests normalized to urine creatinine (UPCR and UACR) are often obtained in the post–kidney transplant setting. These can be used for proteinuria screening, assessing the response to therapy, or monitoring for the recurrence of native kidney disease. Both of these tests correlate well with the 24-hour urine protein in general, but they are affected by urine creatinine concentrations (the denominator). For example, in a patient with low muscle mass, urine creatinine will be low and therefore urine proteinuria will be overestimated. In a muscular person with a high urine creatinine, the proteinuria may be underestimated. Additionally, urine protein excretion can vary in certain settings, including exercise and posture, and there are normal slight variations on a day-to-day basis.

Obtaining a timed 24-hour urine collection for protein is theoretically the best test for quantifying proteinuria. The problem is that this test is cumbersome for the patient. Not uncommonly there is an overcollection or undercollection, making the test unreliable. We recommend using the spot UPCR or UACR for routine clinical monitoring. A timed collection can be obtained on less-frequent intervals to validate the spot urine findings or quantify the amount of proteinuria if new proteinuria is detected with the UPCR or UACR.

Electrolytes

Electrolyte abnormalities are common post–kidney transplant, especially in the early period, and thus frequent electrolyte monitoring is recommended. Hyperkalemia is common electrolyte abnormality post–kidney transplant that is likely medication induced, but exacerbated by allograft dysfunction. Calcineurin inhibitors, trimethoprim-sulfamethoxazole, beta blockers, angiotensin enzyme inhibitors, and angiotensin receptor blockers all contribute to hyperkalemia. Hypomagnesemia is also common in the post–kidney transplant period. Multiple factors likely contribute, including calcineurin inhibitor use, proton pump inhibitors, diabetes, diarrhea, and other electrolyte abnormalities. Calcineurin inhibitors (both tacrolimus and cyclosporine) are known to cause renal magnesium wasting, whereas proton pump inhibitors reduce magnesium absorption in the gastrointestinal tract. Metabolic acidosis can result from impaired allograft function, impaired renal bicarbonate handling, and calcineurin toxicity. Last, up to 90% of kidney transplant recipients have an abnormality in calcium or phosphorus posttransplant. This is often the result of metabolic bone disease, but medications such as tacrolimus can also contribute by increasing urinary phosphorus loss.

Immunosuppression Monitoring

Dosing adjustments for immunosuppressive medications, including calcineurin (tacrolimus and cyclosporine) and mammalian target of rapamycin (mTOR) inhibitors (sirolimus and everolimus) are generally determined by drug levels and patient characteristics (risk of rejection and/or infection). Calcineurin inhibitor blood levels need to be followed very closely early posttransplant until the target levels have reached steady state. At a minimum, drug target levels should also be measured whenever there is a dose adjustment, change in patient status, initiation of medication that interferes with immunosuppressive drug levels, or decline in kidney function. Tacrolimus, cyclosporine, and mTOR inhibitors are usually monitored using a 12-hour trough. Measuring a 2-hour post-dose peak or abbreviated area under the curve (AUC) is acceptable for cyclosporine testing. Some centers also routinely monitor mycophenolate levels by using a 12-hour trough or AUC, but because they are less reliable, this is not a universal practice.

SCREENING FOR COMMON COMORBID CONDITIONS AND MEDICATION SIDE EFFECTS

An important aspect of following kidney transplant patients long-term is screening for and managing the comorbid conditions that are often associated with chronic kidney disease and/or the complex immunosuppressive medication regimen. Cardiovascular disease, diabetes, obesity, metabolic bone disease, hematologic abnormalities, malignancy, and infection are all associated with kidney transplantation and immunosuppressive medications. The management of these conditions and side effects is essential for the health of the kidney allograft as well as the patient.

Cardiovascular disease is a major cause of death in kidney transplant recipients. In part, this is related to the comorbid conditions that led to kidney failure initially, but chronic kidney disease and posttransplant complications are associated with cardiovascular disease. Laboratory monitoring does not play a major role in identifying cardiovascular disease itself, but is important to identify risk factors such as hyperlipidemia and diabetes. A lipid profile should be obtained in all adults who have undergone transplantation.[11,12] A follow-up lipid profile is not recommended based on updated KDIGO (Kidney Disease: Improving Global Outcomes) hyperlipidemia guidelines after the initiation of lipid-lowering therapy unless there is concern about adherence to statin therapy or concern about the presence of new secondary reasons for hyperlipidemia.[11,12]

The incidence of posttransplant diabetes has been reported to range from 7% up to 46%[13,14] in kidney transplant recipients. Steroids and tacrolimus are important contributors, but other factors, including the propensity for weight gain after transplantation, play a role in the development of glucose intolerance posttransplant. With improved kidney function, insulin is metabolized and excreted more rapidly and thus even patients who had well-controlled diabetes pretransplant may find that their hyperglycemia is difficult to control posttransplant. According to KDIGO guidelines, all nondiabetic kidney transplant recipients should have fasting plasma glucose, oral glucose tolerance testing, and/or HbA1c at least weekly for 4 weeks, every 3 months for a year, and annually, thereafter.[15]

Metabolic bone disease following the kidney transplant results from a combination of preexisting hyperparathyroidism and osteoporosis and is associated with significant morbidity and mortality. Routine calcium, phosphorus, 25 hydroxyvitamin D, and parathyroid hormone are important laboratory screening tests. At minimum, calcium and phosphorus should be obtained weekly if not more frequently immediately posttransplantation until stable. Parathyroid hormone also should be obtained at baseline posttransplant and at regular intervals based on the degree of allograft function. Transplant recipients with excellent allograft function (chronic kidney disease [CKD] stages 1–3T) can be monitored every 6 to 12 months, whereas recipients with allograft dysfunction (CKD stage 5) should have laboratory monitoring for hyperparathyroidism every 1 to 3 months. Vitamin D (inactive – 25 hydroxyvitamin D) testing should be obtained at baseline and as needed based on other metabolic bone disease parameters.

Hematologic complications, especially anemia and leukopenia, are associated with immunosuppressive medications and reduced allograft function. Regular monitoring of complete blood counts (CBCs) are important for identification. A CBC should be checked almost daily until hospital dismissal following the transplant and then 2 to 3 times per week for the first month, weekly up to 3 months posttransplant, and monthly thereafter for the first year posttransplant. At minimum, a CBC should be checked annually in posttransplant patients.

INFECTIOUS DISEASE SURVEILLANCE

Effective immunosuppressive regimens are important to reduce the incidence of acute rejection, but this must be balanced with the transplant recipients' susceptibility to infection. Vaccination and prophylactic antimicrobial strategies have been successful at reducing opportunistic infection in transplant recipients, but routine monitoring for common posttransplant infections remains important, especially because the typical signs and symptoms of infection can be diminished in immunocompromised hosts. Monitoring for asymptomatic disease informs decisions regarding immunosuppression management to prevent more infectious disease complications.

Urinary tract infection is the most common infection after kidney transplantation, accounting for 45% of infectious complications.[16,17] Approximately 25% of kidney transplant recipients experience a urinary tract infection within the first year posttransplant.[18] This is important because urinary tract infections are associated with rejection, allograft loss, and patient mortality.[18] Unfortunately, there is a paucity of data regarding the role of screening for urinary tract infection. In part this may be related to unnecessary antibiotic administration that can lead to microbial resistance and medication side effects. The Infectious Disease Community of Practice as part of the American Society of Transplantation recommends that screening for asymptomatic bacteriuria be limited to the first 1 to 3 months posttransplant or at the time of elevations in creatinine.[19]

To reduce the morbidity and mortality of cytomegalovirus (CMV) disease, laboratory monitoring with CMV nucleic acid testing to detect viral load is important, especially in CMV-negative transplant recipients who receive an organ from a CMV-positive recipient. Cytomegalovirus nucleic acid testing is also recommended weekly to monitor response to therapy in patients with a known CMV infection. Either universal antiviral therapy or preemptive therapy strategies are used for CMV disease prevention. In the preemptive strategy approach, patients are monitored for CMV viremia at regular intervals (often weekly). Viral monitoring may also play a role after completion of an antiviral prophylaxis strategy. Regular monitoring (ie, weekly) of CMV for 8 to 12 weeks after discontinuation of antiviral prophylaxis is a consideration, but this has not been well studied.[20]

Transplant recipients who are seronegative for Epstein-Barr virus (EBV) who receive an organ from a seropositive donor are at risk for EBV viremia and potentially posttransplant lymphoproliferative disease. Thus, monitoring for EBV viremia with EBV nucleic acid testing is recommended frequently in the first year posttransplant or after rejection treatment in high-risk kidney transplant recipients.[15,21]

BK polyomavirus is not associated with systemic disease, but is associated with nephropathy and allograft loss. This disease most commonly occurs in the first year posttransplant. Because this disease is completely asymptomatic, laboratory monitoring is essential to avoid allograft dysfunction. KDIGO recommends that BK testing with plasma nucleic acid monthly for the first 3 to 6 months posttransplant, then every 3 months until the end of the first year posttransplant.[12] BK testing also should be considered whenever there is an unexplained reduction in allograft function.

DONOR-SPECIFIC ANTIBODY TESTING

De novo donor-specific antibody (dnDSA) is a major risk factor for chronic antibody-mediated rejection and allograft loss.[22–26] Depending on the cohort studied, the incidence of dnDSA varies from 6.2% to 27.8%,[23–25,27–30] and approximately one-quarter of allografts fail within 3 years of dnDSA detection.[24] For these reasons, detection of dnDSA by routine surveillance testing or at the time of allograft dysfunction has major prognostic value. However, the available therapies to reduce dnDSA or the accompanying antibody-mediated rejection have questionable effectiveness, and thus one could debate the benefit in routine donor-specific antibody (DSA) testing.

Even if effective therapy to reliably reduce DSA is not available, a patient with newly identified DSA should be managed differently. The main risk factor for dnDSA is inadequate immunosuppression either prescribed by the physician or nonadherence by the patient. In either case, the patient's immunosuppressive regimen should be optimized and a less complicated immunosuppressive regimen could be considered. Patients with dnDSA should also be monitored more frequently. This is especially important in patients who are prone to medication nonadherence, but this is important for all patients with newly identified dnDSA. Given the increased rate of allograft dysfunction and loss, the frequency of face-to-face visits, renal function, and proteinuria monitoring should be increased. Transplant recipients with dnDSA with a rapid decline in kidney function also can be referred for transplant reevaluation. Last, a transplant kidney biopsy should be strongly considered for all patients with dnDSA, because not only is dnDSA associated with antibody-mediated rejection, it is also associated with T-cell–mediated rejection, which can be often effectively treated.[23,31]

The available testing for DSA has important limitations, and thus the results of DSA testing need to be carefully interpreted in context. Additionally, repeat DSA testing is to confirm the persistence of DSA because patients with transient DSA positivity have improved outcomes.[31] A discussion regarding the interpretation of commercially available and investigational DSA testing follows.

The Solid-Phase Single-Antigen Bead Assay

The current fluorescent-based solid-phase assays are more commonly used to detect dnDSA. These tests are able to distinguish up to 100 different micro particles or beads with different HLA antigens. Multi-antigen or phenotypic beads contain antigens from a single cell line (Class I and Class II), whereas each single-antigen bead (SAB) contains a purified single HLA antigen.[32] The transplant recipient's serum is incubated with the solid-phase platform (multi-antigen or single-antigen beads) and a fluorescent-conjugated anti-human immunoglobulin (Ig)G, which binds to alloantibody bound to its targeted antigen. In both cases, the beads contain a distinctive ratio of varied fluorochromes that provides a unique signal recognized by Luminex technology.[32] If the multi-antigen beads used for screening are positive, we suggest doing SABs to precisely identify the donor-specific antibody.

The SAB output is mean fluorescence intensity (MFI), which is a semiquantitative measure of the amount and/or avidity of antibody (total IgG – all subclasses combined).

However, the assay is approved by the Food and Drug Administration only as a qualitative assay (negative or positive). Determining a negative SAB result is often the single most important aspect of alloantibody testing, yet this can be difficult because results are not dichotomous and can vary based on laboratory conditions. The MFI threshold to differentiate negative and positive also varies among transplant centers.

The problem with relying on the MFI alone is that the MFI result is only semiquantitative and prone to both false-positive and false-negative results. False-positive results can occur if antibodies bind to a denatured form of antigen.[33–35] Additionally, high levels of anti-HLA antibody with strong affinity and avidity can saturate the beads or interfere with alloantibody binding leading to results that are lower than expected for a particular antigenic specificity. This is referred to as the prozone or hook effect. External substances such as IgM antibody,[36] intravenous immunoglobulin, antithymocyte globulin,[37] immune complexes, complement,[38,39] or nonspecific binding of external substances can also interfere with antigen/antibody binding leading to this phenomenon.[40,41] The prozone or hook effect does not necessarily affect all antigen specificities for a particular patient at one time. Serum treatment with EDTA/dithiothreitol, heat, or hypotonic dialysis treatment[39,40] can mitigate this effect somewhat, but these treatments can also nonuniformly dilute the sample, making the MFI results less reproducible. The most reliable way to recognize prozone is to do a serum dilution and repeat the assay. If the MFI does not decrease in a linear fashion as expected, a prozone effect should be suspected.

Donor-Specific Antibody Titer

Because the SAB test results are semiquantitative, to reliably determine the change in antibody level, with or without treatment, serial dilutions are needed to obtain the DSA titer. The problem is that obtaining the DSA titer requires the performance of multiple SAB tests, and thus it is expensive and labor intensive. The advantage of obtaining the DSA titer as compared with performing one dilution to identify prozone has not been shown, and thus we do not routinely recommend obtaining DSA titer outside of research purposes to determine if a particular therapy is effective for DSA reduction. Obtaining DSA titer will likely become more important in the future if effective therapy to reduce DSA becomes available and a reduction in DSA titer is shown to be associated with improved outcomes.

Complement-Binding Donor-Specific Antibody

Complement activation is an important mechanism by which DSA leads to allograft damage, and this activation begins by antibody binding of C1q.[42] Downstream, C3 is cleaved leaving C3d. Commercially available modified SAB tests have been developed to specifically detect C1q and C3d binding.[43,44] DSA with C1q and/or C3d binding positivity is associated with the development of antibody-mediated rejection (AMR) and allograft loss,[44–46] and some groups routinely use these tests to distinguish the most deleterious DSA. However, the presence of C1q or C3d binding antibodies is also associated with DSA MFI and antibody titer[47–49]; therefore, it remains unknown whether C1q positivity is any more predictive of AMR or graft loss than MFI or antibody titer.[41,47,50] Thus, testing for C1q or C3d binding is not yet universally performed.

Immunoglobulin Subclasses

Commercially available SABs are used to detect total IgG rather than IgG subclasses. This is relevant because each subclass has a differing role in the immune response and varied effector functions (for example, to bind the Fc receptor or activate complement).[51] It is possible that specific subclass profiles may be predictive of the development of AMR or allograft loss than total IgG. IgG subclass characterization is now performed in the research setting using a modified SAB assay in which the conventional phycoerythrin-conjugated anti-human IgG is replaced with an IgG subclass-specific anti-human IgG.[52] Of the 4 subclasses, IgG1/IgG3 has the strongest ability to bind complement. Emerging evidence suggests that DSA of the IgG3 subclass is particularly deleterious to the renal allografts.[52–59] However, studies of IgG subclasses in transplantation are limited because few groups have examined complete IgG subclass characterization (IgG1–IgG4) serially. The complexity of studying IgG subclasses is overwhelming, but provides clues about the pathogenicity of certain DSA and the immune response.

SURVEILLANCE ALLOGRAFT BIOPSY

Kidney allograft biopsies are most often performed in the setting of allograft dysfunction or proteinuria; however, some centers routinely perform surveillance allograft biopsies, because as discussed previously, measures of kidney function, such as creatinine, are a relatively insensitive and late indication of allograft pathology.[60] Markers of allograft function are also nonspecific, and kidney transplant allografts fail for a variety of reasons.[61] Most surveillance biopsy studies have focused on identifying rejection, but surveillance biopsies provide information about subclinical native disease recurrence and metabolic complications posttransplant, such as diabetes mellitus. Several studies have shown that findings on surveillance biopsies have prognostic value, but it remains unclear whether routine surveillance biopsies lead to improved long-term allograft survival.

Surveillance Biopsy Findings

The incidence of subclinical rejection at very early time points less than 6 months posttransplant ranges from as low as 2.6% up to approximately 50.0% depending on donor and recipient characteristics, induction, and maintenance immunosuppression.[62,63] In the setting of induction with T-cell depletion and maintenance immunosuppression with tacrolimus and mycophenolate mofetil, subclinical rejection is very low at 2.6%.[62] Subclinical rejection is important to identify because several studies have shown that when left untreated, interstitial inflammation is associated with the development of interstitial fibrosis and tubular atrophy.[63–65] Inflammation present on the biopsy that is below the threshold of "rejection" found on protocol biopsies within the first 6 months posttransplant is associated with reduced allograft function at 1 and 2 years posttransplant.[66] Findings other than subclinical rejection identified on early surveillance biopsies are associated with allograft function and failure. Fibrosis, inflammation, and chronic glomerulopathy identified on 1-year surveillance biopsies was predictive of allograft function decline and graft failure, which was independent of graft function at the time of biopsy.[67]

Surveillance biopsies at time points beyond 1 year also provide important clues about why allografts eventually fail.[61] Major histologic abnormalities were found in most of a single-center cohort of kidney transplant recipients who underwent surveillance biopsies at 5 and 10 years posttransplant.[68] At 5 years, 54% of this cohort had evidence of a major histologic abnormality, including chronic transplant glomerulopathy, global glomerulosclerosis greater than 20%, mesangial sclerosis, arteriolar hyalinosis, or other chronic Banff score ≥2.[68] By 10 years posttransplant, 82% of allografts had a major histologic abnormality, and 48% had more than 1 major histologic abnormality.[68] In high-risk patients with preexisting or de novo DSA, subclinical active and chronic AMR is common.[23,31,69]

The central question is whether finding subclinical histologic abnormalities on surveillance biopsy leads to a change in management that ultimately leads to improved allograft survival.[70] Furthermore, is the incidence of a reversible finding high enough to warrant surveillance biopsies in low-risk renal transplant recipients? A small randomized control trial has shown that protocol biopsy and treatment of subclinical rejection at 2 to 3 months posttransplant was associated with reduced interstitial fibrosis at month 6 and improved allograft function at 24 months compared with a control group that did not undergo protocol biopsy.[71] Other than this randomized controlled trial performed before the current era of immunosuppression therapy, no randomized controlled trials have been shown to demonstrate that surveillance biopsy leads to improved allograft survival.[72]

Who to Biopsy and When?

No consensus about the timing or ideal patient population for surveillance biopsy has been reached by the transplant community; thus, surveillance biopsy protocols are transplant center specific. KDIGO suggests a kidney allograft biopsy when there is persistent unexplained decrease in allograft function, but no recommendations are provided for or against surveillance biopsy.[15] Surveillance biopsies can be performed in all kidney transplant recipients or only those at high risk for underlying pathology (ie, native kidney disease with propensity for recurrence, BK viremia, or DSA). A survey of transplant centers in the United States showed that 17% of centers perform surveillance biopsies on all patients, whereas another 21% of centers perform biopsies in high-risk patients only.[73] The most common time points for biopsy are 3 and 12 months. No difference in observed to expected allograft survival at 1 and 3 years posttransplant was found among transplant centers that did or did not perform surveillance biopsy.[73]

Disadvantages of Surveillance Biopsy

The disadvantage of surveillance biopsy is complications such as bleeding or damage to surrounding organs, but these complications are rare.[62,74] Protocol biopsies are associated with fewer complications than indication or native kidney biopsy. The incidence of major complication, including the need for blood transfusion or catheterization has been reported to be from 0.4% to 1.0%. Allograft biopsies are also expensive,[62] but this must be balanced with the potential that they lead to improved outcomes because returning to dialysis is also expensive. Other issues to consider include sampling error and nonspecific histologic lesions. Although not studied, surveillance biopsies could also theoretically lead clinicians to overtreat subclinical lesions.

Although practice patterns regarding surveillance biopsy are not standard, all would agree that it is critical to minimize the risk of the biopsy. This includes ensuring that the patient is normotensive, has normal coagulation parameters and is off of anticoagulation including aspirin, does not have anatomic abnormalities, does not have a urinary tract infection, and is not pregnant.

SUMMARY

Posttransplant monitoring is important to maintain the health of the transplant recipient and the renal allograft. Although few randomized controlled trials have been performed in transplant to inform the optimal monitoring strategy, a general consensus about general laboratory monitoring, including kidney function and infectious disease surveillance, has been reached. Surveillance biopsies and testing for DSA clearly have prognostic value, but it remains unclear whether the use of these tests for surveillance purposes only leads to improved allograft survival.

REFERENCES

1. Rule AD, Bergstralh EJ, Slezak JM, et al. Glomerular filtration rate estimated by cystatin C among different clinical presentations. Kidney Int 2006;69(2):399–405.
2. Le Bricon T, Thervet E, Froissart M, et al. Plasma cystatin C is superior to 24-h creatinine clearance and plasma creatinine for estimation of glomerular filtration rate 3 months after kidney transplantation. Clin Chem 2000;46(8 Pt 1):1206–7.
3. Hoek FJ, Kemperman FA, Krediet RT. A comparison between cystatin C, plasma creatinine and the Cockcroft and Gault formula for the estimation of glomerular filtration rate. Nephrol Dial Transplant 2003;18(10):2024–31.
4. Hojs R, Bevc S, Ekart R, et al. Serum cystatin C-based equation compared to serum creatinine-based equations for estimation of glomerular filtration rate in patients with chronic kidney disease. Clin Nephrol 2008;70(1):10–7.
5. Shlipak MG, Wassel Fyr CL, Chertow GM, et al. Cystatin C and mortality risk in the elderly: the health, aging, and body composition study. J Am Soc Nephrol 2006; 17(1):254–61.
6. Shlipak MG, Sarnak MJ, Katz R, et al. Cystatin C and the risk of death and cardiovascular events among elderly persons. N Engl J Med 2005;352(20):2049–60.
7. Torres da Costa ESV, Costalonga EC, Coelho FO, et al. Assessment of kidney function in patients with cancer. Adv Chronic Kidney Dis 2018;25(1):49–56.
8. Manetti L, Pardini E, Genovesi M, et al. Thyroid function differently affects serum cystatin C and creatinine concentrations. J Endocrinol Invest 2005;28(4):346–9.
9. Knight EL, Verhave JC, Spiegelman D, et al. Factors influencing serum cystatin C levels other than renal function and the impact on renal function measurement. Kidney Int 2004;65(4):1416–21.
10. Bokenkamp A, Domanetzki M, Zinck R, et al. Cystatin C serum concentrations underestimate glomerular filtration rate in renal transplant recipients. Clin Chem 1999;45(10):1866–8.
11. Colvin-Adams M, Smithy JM, Heubner BM, et al. OPTN/SRTR 2012 annual data report: heart. Am J Transplant 2014;14(Suppl 1):113–38.
12. Wanner C, Tonelli M, Kidney Disease: Improving Global Outcomes Lipid Guideline Development Work Group Members. KDIGO Clinical Practice Guideline for Lipid Management in CKD: summary of recommendation statements and clinical approach to the patient. Kidney Int 2014;85(6):1303–9.
13. Heisel O, Heisel R, Balshaw R, et al. New onset diabetes mellitus in patients receiving calcineurin inhibitors: a systematic review and meta-analysis. Am J Transplant 2004;4(4):583–95.
14. Cosio FG, Pesavento TE, Osei K, et al. Post-transplant diabetes mellitus: increasing incidence in renal allograft recipients transplanted in recent years. Kidney Int 2001;59(2):732–7.
15. Kasiske BL, Zeier MG, Chapman JR, et al. KDIGO clinical practice guideline for the care of kidney transplant recipients: a summary. Kidney Int 2010;77(4): 299–311.
16. Alangaden GJ, Thyagarajan R, Gruber SA, et al. Infectious complications after kidney transplantation: current epidemiology and associated risk factors. Clin Transplant 2006;20(4):401–9.
17. Chuang P, Parikh CR, Langone A. Urinary tract infections after renal transplantation: a retrospective review at two US transplant centers. Clin Transplant 2005; 19(2):230–5.
18. Abbott KC, Swanson SJ, Richter ER, et al. Late urinary tract infection after renal transplantation in the United States. Am J Kidney Dis 2004;44(2):353–62.

19. Parasuraman R, Julian K, AST Infectious Diseases Community of Practice. Urinary tract infections in solid organ transplantation. Am J Transplant 2013; 13(Suppl 4):327–36.

20. Humar A, Snydman D, AST Infectious Diseases Community of Practice. Cytomegalovirus in solid organ transplant recipients. Am J Transplant 2009;9(Suppl 4):S78–86.

21. Morton M, Coupes B, Roberts SA, et al. Epstein-Barr virus infection in adult renal transplant recipients. Am J Transplant 2014;14(7):1619–29.

22. Terasaki PI, Ozawa M. Predictive value of HLA antibodies and serum creatinine in chronic rejection: results of a 2-year prospective trial. Transplantation 2005;80(9): 1194–7.

23. Wiebe C, Gibson IW, Blydt-Hansen TD, et al. Evolution and clinical pathologic correlations of de novo donor-specific HLA antibody post kidney transplant. Am J Transplant 2012;12(5):1157–67.

24. Everly MJ, Rebellato LM, Haisch CE, et al. Incidence and impact of de novo donor-specific alloantibody in primary renal allografts. Transplantation 2013; 95(3):410–7.

25. Hidalgo LG, Campbell PM, Sis B, et al. De novo donor-specific antibody at the time of kidney transplant biopsy associates with microvascular pathology and late graft failure. Am J Transplant 2009;9(11):2532–41.

26. Hourmant M, Cesbron-Gautier A, Terasaki PI, et al. Frequency and clinical implications of development of donor-specific and non-donor-specific HLA antibodies after kidney transplantation. J Am Soc Nephrol 2005;16(9):2804–12.

27. Wiebe C, Gibson IW, Blydt-Hansen TD, et al. Rates and determinants of progression to graft failure in kidney allograft recipients with de novo donor-specific antibody. Am J Transplant 2015;15(11):2921–30.

28. Cooper JE, Gralla J, Chan L, et al. Clinical significance of post kidney transplant de novo DSA in otherwise stable grafts. Clin Transpl 2011;359–64.

29. DeVos JM, Patel SJ, Burns KM, et al. De novo donor specific antibodies and patient outcomes in renal transplantation. Clin Transpl 2011;351–8.

30. de Kort H, Willicombe M, Brookes P, et al. Microcirculation inflammation associates with outcome in renal transplant patients with de novo donor-specific antibodies. Am J Transplant 2013;13(2):485–92.

31. Schinstock CA, Cosio F, Cheungpasitporn W, et al. The value of protocol biopsies to identify patients with de novo donor-specific antibody at high risk for allograft loss. Am J Transplant 2017;17(6):1574–84.

32. Lachmann N, Todorova K, Schulze H, et al. Luminex((R)) and its applications for solid organ transplantation, hematopoietic stem cell transplantation, and transfusion. Transfus Med Hemother 2013;40(3):182–9.

33. Jacob EK, De Goey SR, Gandhi MJ. Positive virtual crossmatch with negative flow crossmatch results in two cases. Transpl Immunol 2011;25(1):77–81.

34. Visentin J, Guidicelli G, Moreau JF, et al. Deciphering allogeneic antibody response against native and denatured HLA epitopes in organ transplantation. Eur J Immunol 2015;45(7):2111–21.

35. Dias AL, Hashmi S, Hogan W, et al. The 'HLA conundrum in bone marrow transplantation': correct interpretation of anti-HLA antibodies in haploidentical donor selection. Bone Marrow Transplant 2017;52(6):902–4.

36. Kosmoliaptsis V, Bradley JA, Peacock S, et al. Detection of immunoglobulin G human leukocyte antigen-specific alloantibodies in renal transplant patients using single-antigen-beads is compromised by the presence of immunoglobulin M

human leukocyte antigen-specific alloantibodies. Transplantation 2009;87(6): 813–20.

37. Gloor JM, Moore SB, Schneider BA, et al. The effect of antithymocyte globulin on anti-human leukocyte antigen antibody detection assays. Transplantation 2007; 84(2):258–64.

38. Visentin J, Vigata M, Daburon S, et al. Deciphering complement interference in anti-human leukocyte antigen antibody detection with flow beads assays. Transplantation 2014;98(6):625–31.

39. Schnaidt M, Weinstock C, Jurisic M, et al. HLA antibody specification using single-antigen beads—a technical solution for the prozone effect. Transplantation 2011;92(5):510–5.

40. Zachary AA, Lucas DP, Detrick B, et al. Naturally occurring interference in Luminex assays for HLA-specific antibodies: characteristics and resolution. Hum Immunol 2009;70(7):496–501.

41. Tambur AR, Herrera ND, Haarberg KM, et al. Assessing antibody strength: comparison of MFI, C1q, and titer information. Am J Transplant 2015;15(9):2421–30.

42. Stegall MD, Chedid MF, Cornell LD. The role of complement in antibody-mediated rejection in kidney transplantation. Nat Rev Nephrol 2012;8(11):670–8.

43. Chen G, Sequeira F, Tyan DB. Novel C1q assay reveals a clinically relevant subset of human leukocyte antigen antibodies independent of immunoglobulin G strength on single antigen beads. Hum Immunol 2011;72(10):849–58.

44. Sicard A, Ducreux S, Rabeyrin M, et al. Detection of C3d-binding donor-specific anti-HLA antibodies at diagnosis of humoral rejection predicts renal graft loss. J Am Soc Nephrol 2015;26(2):457–67.

45. Loupy A, Lefaucheur C, Vernerey D, et al. Complement-binding anti-HLA antibodies and kidney-allograft survival. N Engl J Med 2013;369(13):1215–26.

46. Baid-Agrawal S, Lachmann N, Budde K. Complement-binding anti-HLA antibodies and kidney transplantation. N Engl J Med 2014;370(1):84.

47. Zeevi A, Lunz J, Feingold B, et al. Persistent strong anti-HLA antibody at high titer is complement binding and associated with increased risk of antibody-mediated rejection in heart transplant recipients. J Heart Lung Transplant 2013;32(1): 98–105.

48. Schaub S, Honger G, Koller MT, et al. Determinants of C1q binding in the single antigen bead assay. Transplantation 2014;98(4):387–93.

49. Moreno Gonzales MA, Mitema DG, Smith BH, et al. Comparison between total IgG, C1q, and C3d single antigen bead assays in detecting class I complement-binding Anti-HLA antibodies. Transplant Proc 2017;49(9):2031–5.

50. Gandhi M, Degoey S, Henderson N, et al. C1q single antigen bead assay only detects high titer/avidity class-I anti HLA antibodies detected by single antigen beads. Hum Immunol 2014;75:73.

51. Nimmerjahn F, Ravetch JV. Divergent immunoglobulin G subclass activity through selective Fc receptor binding. Science 2005;310(5753):1510–2.

52. Kaneku H, O'Leary JG, Taniguchi M, et al. Donor-specific human leukocyte antigen antibodies of the immunoglobulin G3 subclass are associated with chronic rejection and graft loss after liver transplantation. Liver Transpl 2012;18(8): 984–92.

53. Taner T, Gandhi MJ, Sanderson SO, et al. Prevalence, course and impact of HLA donor-specific antibodies in liver transplantation in the first year. Am J Transplant 2012;12(6):1504–10.

54. O'Leary JG, Klintmalm GB. Impact of donor-specific antibodies on results of liver transplantation. Curr Opin Organ Transplant 2013;18(3):279–84.

55. O'Leary JG, Demetris AJ, Friedman LS, et al. The role of donor-specific HLA alloantibodies in liver transplantation. Am J Transplant 2014;14(4):779–87.
56. Everly MJ, Rebellato LM, Haisch CE, et al. Impact of IgM and IgG3 anti-HLA alloantibodies in primary renal allograft recipients. Transplantation 2014;97(5): 494–501.
57. Schinstock CR, Cosio S, Cornell F, et al. Donor-specific alloantibody after positive crossmatch kidney transplant with eculizumab: correlation with transplant glomerulopathy and graft failure [abstract]. Am J Transplant 2015;15(suppl 3).
58. Freitas MC, Rebellato LM, Ozawa M, et al. The role of immunoglobulin-G subclasses and C1q in de novo HLA-DQ donor-specific antibody kidney transplantation outcomes. Transplantation 2013;95(9):1113–9.
59. Lefaucheur C, Viglietti D, Bentlejewski C, et al. IgG donor-specific anti-human HLA antibody subclasses and kidney allograft antibody-mediated injury. J Am Soc Nephrol 2016;27(1):293–304.
60. Yilmaz S, Isik I, Afrouzian M, et al. Evaluating the accuracy of functional biomarkers for detecting histological changes in chronic allograft nephropathy. Transpl Int 2007;20(7):608–15.
61. El-Zoghby ZM, Stegall MD, Lager DJ, et al. Identifying specific causes of kidney allograft loss. Am J Transplant 2009;9(3):527–35.
62. Gloor JM, Cohen AJ, Lager DJ, et al. Subclinical rejection in tacrolimus-treated renal transplant recipients. Transplantation 2002;73(12):1965–8.
63. Nankivell BJ, Borrows RJ, Fung CL, et al. Natural history, risk factors, and impact of subclinical rejection in kidney transplantation. Transplantation 2004;78(2): 242–9.
64. Nankivell BJ, Fenton-Lee CA, Kuypers DR, et al. Effect of histological damage on long-term kidney transplant outcome. Transplantation 2001;71(4):515–23.
65. Choi BS, Shin MJ, Shin SJ, et al. Clinical significance of an early protocol biopsy in living-donor renal transplantation: ten-year experience at a single center. Am J Transplant 2005;5(6):1354–60.
66. Mengel M, Gwinner W, Schwarz A, et al. Infiltrates in protocol biopsies from renal allografts. Am J Transplant 2007;7(2):356–65.
67. Cosio FG, Grande JP, Wadei H, et al. Predicting subsequent decline in kidney allograft function from early surveillance biopsies. Am J Transplant 2005;5(10): 2464–72.
68. Stegall MD, Cornell LD, Park WD, et al. Renal allograft histology at 10 years after transplantation in the tacrolimus era: evidence of pervasive chronic injury. Am J Transplant 2018;18(1):180–8.
69. Parajuli S, Reville PK, Ellis TM, et al. Utility of protocol kidney biopsies for de novo donor-specific antibodies. Am J Transplant 2017;17(12):3210–8.
70. Rush D. Protocol transplant biopsies: an underutilized tool in kidney transplantation. Clin J Am Soc Nephrol 2006;1(1):138–43.
71. Rush D, Nickerson P, Gough J, et al. Beneficial effects of treatment of early subclinical rejection: a randomized study. J Am Soc Nephrol 1998;9(11):2129–34.
72. Rush D, Arlen D, Boucher A, et al. Lack of benefit of early protocol biopsies in renal transplant patients receiving TAC and MMF: a randomized study. Am J Transplant 2007;7(11):2538–45.
73. Mehta R, Cherikh W, Sood P, et al. Kidney allograft surveillance biopsy practices across US transplant centers: a UNOS survey. Clin Transplant 2017;31(5).
74. Schwarz A, Gwinner W, Hiss M, et al. Safety and adequacy of renal transplant protocol biopsies. Am J Transplant 2005;5(8):1992–6.

Recent Advancements in the Assessment of Renal Transplant Dysfunction with an Emphasis on Microarray Molecular Diagnostics

Meagan Barner, CHS[a,1], Jenefer DeKoning, PhD[a,1],
Zahra Kashi, PhD[a,*], Phillip Halloran, MD, PhD[b,c]

KEYWORDS

- Molecular diagnostics • Renal transplant • T-cell-mediated rejection (TCMR)
- Antibody-mediated rejection (ABMR) • Microarray • Molecular microscope

KEY POINTS

- The ability to accurately diagnose dysfunction in renal transplants is critical for treatment.
- Conventional assessment methods are insensitive (serum creatinine, eGFR), of limited use (C4d and DSA), and often nonspecific (various histologic lesions). In addition, histology is prone to poor interobserver agreement.
- Noninvasive biomarker testing has yet to show enough utility to replace the kidney biopsy as the reference material for diagnosis.
- The Molecular Microscope diagnostic system provides gene expression data that have been validated against conventional biopsy assessments.

CURRENT TRANSPLANT MONITORING

Transplantation has been a life-changing therapy for many patients who have end-stage renal disease. Although the field of transplantation has come a long way, and there are a number of positive trends in allograft survival, long-term graft survival

Disclosure Statement: Dr P. Halloran holds shares in and is CEO of Transcriptome Sciences Inc, a company with an interest in molecular diagnostics.
[a] Kashi Clinical Laboratories, 10101 Southwest Barbur Boulevard Suite 200, Portland, OR 97219, USA; [b] Division of Nephrology and Transplant Immunology, Department of Medicine, University of Alberta, Alberta Transplant Applied Genomics Center, 250 Heritage Medical Research Centre, Edmonton, Alberta T6G 2S2, Canada; [c] Transcriptome Sciences Inc, Edmonton, Alberta, Canada
[1] First 2 authors share first authorship.
* Corresponding author.
E-mail address: zkashi@kashilab.com

continues to be an issue.[1,2] More effective tools are needed to detect the presence, and diagnose the causes, of allograft dysfunction. In particular, the ability to determine if dysfunction is due to antibody-mediated rejection (ABMR), T-cell–mediated rejection (TCMR), or a combination of both, is vital, as ABMR is the leading cause of kidney transplant failure.[3] A correct diagnosis is critical for a clinician to determine the best course of treatment and immunosuppressive regimen for the patient.

The current standards for monitoring kidney transplant function are serum creatinine and estimated glomerular filtration rate (eGFR). However, it has been shown that these are relatively insensitive markers, as they require significant global injury to the kidney before a measurable change can be observed, and these biomarkers are also influenced by multiple nonimmunological factors.[4] Additionally, subclinical cases of rejection are most often not detected by these tests. Histologic evaluation, as well, is not optimal in the diagnosis of rejection, as it relies on nonspecific lesions. For example, in the case of ABMR, microcirculation changes, fibrosis, and arterial fibrous intimal thickening also occur in other conditions, such as TCMR and glomerulonephritis (GN).[5]

Other histopathology criteria that are diagnostic of ABMR include C4d staining and donor-specific antibodies (DSAs), but both of these methods have a number of limitations.[6] For example, C4d has long been considered a marker for antibody injury. However, we now know that more than half of patients with ABMR have significant microcirculatory inflammation, but are still C4d-negative.[7] Due to the prevalence of C4d-negative ABMR cases, and the assay's low sensitivity and poor reproducibility, the Banff 2013 classification scheme was updated to include analysis of gene expression markers of endothelial injury in the biopsy.[8]

Similarly, there are several challenges with HLA antibody testing. For example, the multiplex bead array assays have inherent limitations that include signal inhibition in the presence of intrinsic or extrinsic factors, oversaturation of single-antigen beads and binding of denatured or cryptic epitopes that are not clinically relevant.[9] Additionally, not all DSAs are equivalent in their association with distinct outcomes and injury phenotypes. Clearly time course, kinetics, and properties of DSA fluctuate. These, along with lack of available DSA data at the time of biopsy, make diagnoses complex. Furthermore, there is a need for comprehensive HLA typing of recipient and donor to determine presence of HLA-DSA and its specificity at the allelic level.

Although ABMR is more likely to lead to graft failure, the correct diagnosis of TCMR in kidney transplants still remains critical in the differential diagnosis of graft dysfunction. The biopsy diagnosis of TCMR is based on Banff guidelines for histologic lesions, including interstitial infiltrate, tubulitis, and intimal arteritis.[6] It is known that it is difficult to assess TCMR lesions in scarred tissue, creating false negatives. It is also known that the interstitial inflammation and tubulitis lesions are nonspecific and found in other conditions, such as acute kidney injury (AKI) and progressive renal diseases, creating the potential for false positives.[10] Furthermore, many biopsies are assigned the ambiguous "borderline" designation because of poor interobserver agreements and lack of clinical reproducibility.[11] Equally confounding, many cases of ABMR in kidney allografts, particularly late ABMR associated with de novo DSAs, can present as mixed ABMR and TCMR.[5] TCMR is often an indication of nonadherence, which is a major risk for graft loss, at least some of which is due to later development of DSA and ABMR.

Noninvasive biomarker testing is an obvious attractive choice for any patient disease monitoring when possible, and several studies have provided evidence to support urine for the sample source in kidney transplant rejection monitoring.[12] Chemokines CXCL10 and CXCL9 were found to be elevated in urine up to 30 days before an episode of acute rejection, and importantly, antirejection treatment resulted in a decrease in their levels. Similarly, urinary transcripts for cytotoxic cell products like perforin and granzyme B are found to be increased in patients with rejection as opposed to nonrejection states.

The use of peripheral blood gene expression profiles as a minimally invasive means to circumvent the need for biopsy also has been extensively studied. Several products are commercially available or soon to be commercially available, including TruGraf, kSort, and Allosure. TruGraf measures expression levels and is intended to be used to monitor stable grafts and to provide early detection of grafts that may develop rejection.[4] kSort uses quantitative real-time polymerase chain reaction to measure expression of 17 genes to provide a risk score for acute rejection, whereas Allosure uses donor-derived cell-free DNA levels to discriminate between any rejection and no rejection.[13,14] The aforementioned tests discriminate only between rejection and nonrejection, and do not provide a complete substitute for histology.

Therefore, given these limitations and the current state of the art, urine and blood biomarkers are not suitable replacements for kidney transplant biopsy in typing and grading renal allograft rejection. Biopsies still remain the gold standard for rejection diagnoses in kidney transplantation. It is also mandatory to constantly adjust our diagnostic standards to reflect current immunologic knowledge. In transplant medicine, molecular profiling strategies using microarrays have shown promise as a new dimension for assessing transplant biopsies.[9] This technology allows for more objective, quantitative, biology-based measurements than conventional histopathology-based diagnoses, and promises a more clinically relevant diagnostic depiction of the rejection processes, providing clinicians more confidence in their clinical management decisions.

INTRODUCTION OF THE MOLECULAR MICROSCOPE

Although molecular profiling of diseased kidneys has been reported by a number of different laboratories over the past several years, a reliable clinical molecular test capable of characterizing and predicting kidney transplant rejection was still lacking. Therefore, the Alberta Transplant Applied Genomics Center (ATAGC), led by Dr Philip Halloran, began the development of a comprehensive system they called the Molecular Microscope (MMDx), which uses computer algorithms based on gene expression data to test kidney biopsies for rejection and injury. The MMDx system uses total RNA extracted from biopsies with Applied Biosystems (Foster City, CA) 3′ IVT PLUS Kits to prepare complementary RNA (cRNA) for gene expression profiling. After the cRNA product is purified and fragmented, it is hybridized to an Applied Biosystems Gene-Chip 3′ Expression Array.[15] The hybridized array is then washed and stained with a streptavidin-phycoerythrin conjugate before being read by a scanner. The Applied Biosystems software automatically analyzes the image produced by the scanner and derives a single intensity value for each probe set and these data undergo a secondary analysis in the MMDx software package developed by ATAGC.[15]

The development of the MMDx system initially required the investigation of genes of interest in various experimental systems, including cell lines, mouse models, and human biopsies.[9] These investigations resulted in annotated lists of gene sets referred to as pathogenesis-based transcript sets (PBTs).[9,16] The PBTs have been used by ATAGC to assign functions to gene lists created when comparing gene expression in disease states and to define groups of biopsies.[9] Although the PBTs are not used to provide a diagnosis, they do provide an understanding of the biological pathways impacted by the disease state of the biopsy.[9]

ATAGC derived the microarray probe sets related to rejection and injury using association analysis. From the associations, classifiers were built to predict disease diagnoses, and the severity of various histologic and clinical variables.[9] The classifiers, or weighted equations, are machine-learning algorithms that predict class membership.[9,17] In each case, the molecular profiles of 2 sets of patients were compared: those with, and those without the condition being assessed (ie, patients with ABMR vs those without). Rejection and injury scores are assigned from the classifiers developed from a reference set of biopsies and externally validated on a new set of biopsies.[10,18] To date, patient data comprises a reference set of 1208 fully phenotyped kidney transplant biopsies. As the complex molecular landscape of a posttransplant kidney was further mapped, classifiers were added that differentiate ABMR[19] and TCMR,[20] predict graft loss,[21] and quantify AKI,[22,23] atrophy-fibrosis,[24] and global disturbance.[9] Classifiers were also developed to predict histologic lesions and the probability of DSA-positive status.[15]

Of the 20,000 genes present on the arrays, expression data from 1494 genes associated with allograft rejection, injury, and tissue-specific markers are assessed using the MMDx software package developed by ATAGC.[25] Using standard cross-validation methods, genes that most strongly associate with differences between the 2 sets of patients are used as input for various machine-learning algorithms. These algorithms find patterns of gene expression that reflect maximal separation between the 2 classes. Each algorithm looks at the problem from a slightly different perspective, and consequently, each generates slightly different, but highly correlated predictions. These are combined to obtain more robust predictions for each phenotype. Subsequently, different disease and disease-lesion predictions are combined in a meta-analysis that makes use of all the relevant phenotypes simultaneously.

Continual refinement of the algorithms has led to the incorporation of archetypal analysis to define a set of pure rejection phenotypes that not only gives the probability of nonrejection, TCMR, and mixed rejection, but further delineates ABMR into early-stage, fully developed, and late-stage disease.[26] Using methods such as nearest neighbors, principal component analysis, and archetypal analysis, a determination can be made as to which patients in the existing reference set a new biopsy most closely resembles at the molecular level to assess the probability of various transplant-related disease states.

THE DEVELOPMENT OF THE ANTIBODY-MEDIATED REJECTION CLASSIFIER

Given the importance of accurately diagnosing ABMR in troubled transplants and the difficulty of this diagnosis when using conventional assessment, the development of the ABMR classifier was both critical and involved. Although the first use of the MMDx protocol was to establish a classifier set for estimating the probability of TCMR,[20] the focus of this review is to primarily highlight the seminal findings during the development of an ABMR probability assessment tool using similar classifiers, and the subsequent compilation of all classifiers that resulted in the final MMDx system test result.

The results of the first 403 kidney transplant biopsies used as a reference set to design the ABMR classifiers for the MMDx system were described by Sellarés and colleagues.[20] These biopsies (termed the BFC403 reference set) were collected prospectively from 315 consenting kidney transplant recipients 6 days to 35 years posttransplant. They had been previously characterized by histology and HLA antibody testing using the reference standard classification based on the Banff 2009 classification guidelines, and included both C4d-positive and C4d-negative ABMR cases.[27]

Using MMDx, ABMR scores were assigned to each biopsy with values between 0 and 1.0, with an arbitrary cutoff of 0.2 selected as positive. TCMR was included with the multiple other diseases in the comparator group to allow the algorithm to separate ABMR cases from TCMR or other general features of kidney damage. The resulting scores showed a strong correlation between the microcirculation lesions of ABMR and DSA; such that every biopsy with an ABMR score greater than 0.5 also had DSA or non–donor-specific antibody (NDSA), including both C4d-positive and C4d-negative ABMR cases, and 87% of these had been previously assigned a histology-DSA diagnosis of ABMR by a pathologist.

The relationship between the classifier scores and the diagnosis of ABMR by histology-DSA is demonstrated in **Fig. 1**. The median ABMR score for each biopsy is shown. The statistics for this comparison were as follows: accuracy 85%, sensitivity 67%, specificity 90%, positive predictive value (PPV) 64%, and negative predictive value (NPV) 91%.

One important finding in this study was that the MMDx ABMR score could differentiate between microcirculation abnormalities and general fibrosis, as those biopsies previously diagnosed as "atrophy-fibrosis" received low ABMR scores, with less than 1% receiving scores greater than 0.5.

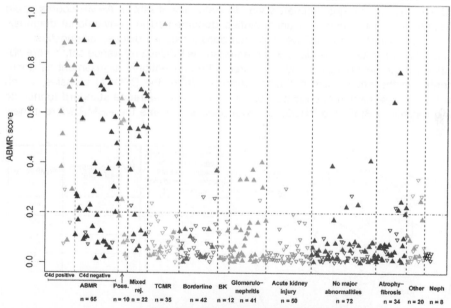

Fig. 1. Relationship between the median ABMR score and the reference standard histology–DSA diagnoses, assigned primarily by the readings of pathologist B as outlined in the Methods section. Ordering within each diagnosis is random. The horizontal line shows the threshold of 0.2 for defining high versus low ABMR scores. The different symbols represent time posttransplantation: early (<1 year: *inverted empty triangles*); and late (>1 year: *solid triangles*). Colors cycle through the diagnostic categories as an aid to separating biopsies close to the vertical partitions between diagnostic stacks. BK, polyoma virus nephropathy; Neph., nephrectomies; Poss., possible ABMR. (*Data from* Sellarés J, Reeve J, Loupy A, et al. Molecular diagnosis of antibody-mediated rejection in human kidney transplants. Am J Transplant 2013;13(4):971–83.)

Fewer than 5% of biopsies were classified as ABMR by conventional histology-DSA, but resulted in low MMDx ABMR scores. Despite these discrepancies, it was demonstrated that for a subset of 245 biopsies, in which diagnostic ABMR microcirculation lesions were observed independently by 3 pathologists, a strong association with the ABMR score was confirmed (G = 0.77–0.81). **Fig. 2** illustrates by Venn diagram that when all 3 pathologists agreed the criteria were met, the mean ABMR score was 0.49, and conversely, the score was 0.09 in biopsies when all 3 agreed the criteria were not met. This strongly suggested that ABMR scores reflect the likelihood of significant agreement among pathologists.

But how did the ABMR score relate to graft survival? Using both the ABMR score and classifications of histologic ABMR, a regression analysis of graft failures was applied to predict death-censored graft survival in their set of 315 biopsies. When the ABMR score was combined with the most significant histologic definition of ABMR (C4d+/–/mixed) in multivariable analysis, it retained its significance. Thus, they concluded that the molecular score can be said to perform at least as well as conventional histologic definitions of ABMR as an independent predictor of graft survival.

To further validate the ABMR score and assess its potential impact on clinical practice, 300 new biopsies (termed the INT300 set) were obtained from 6 centers for use in the International Collaborative Microarray Study (INTERCOM) (clinicaltrials.gov NCT01299168). The goal ultimately was to determine if MMDx ABMR scores could alleviate the all too common uncertainties documented in conventional diagnosis and move toward a more reliable gold standard for kidney disease diagnostics.

ABMR scores, using the classifiers created in the BFC403 reference set,[20] were obtained for the new biopsies and compared with conventional assessment as documented in the prospective pathology reports. Unlike the BFC403 biopsies, which had to be assessed in one location to develop a new reference standard to include C4d-negative ABMR, the INT300 set was used to validate the ABMR score in new

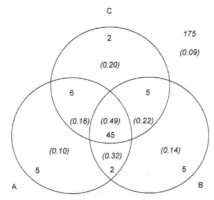

Number of pathologists agreeing that the diagnostic ABMR microcirculation lesions were present	Number of biopsies (total = 245)	ABMR score
3 of 3	45	0.49
2 of 3	13	0.20
1 of 3	12	0.15
0 of 3	175	0.09

Fig. 2. Venn diagram showing the relationship between the molecular ABMR score and the agreement among pathologists that the diagnostic criteria for ABMR were met (in the 245-biopsy subset). The diagnostic criteria used here were the presence of DSA plus one of ptc greater than 1, g >0, or cg >0 (ptc = peritubular capillaritis; g = glomerulitis; cg = transplant glomerulopathy). Numbers in italics and parentheses show the average molecular ABMR score in the biopsies for the corresponding Venn area. Numbers with no parentheses are the number of biopsies. (*Data from* Sellarés J, Reeve J, Loupy A, et al. Molecular diagnosis of antibody-mediated rejection in human kidney transplants. Am J Transplant 2013;13(4):971–83.)

biopsies and to assess its potential impact when used in a variety of established transplant centers.[10]

An important caveat to this study was there was no attempt to "correct" the local pathologists' assessment or perform a central review. Recognizing the importance of C4d-negative ABMR as well as the inherent controversy among experts regarding the criteria for classification of this disease set, the study was designed to capture variability in the data set to reflect actual clinical practice differences between the transplant centers. When there were potentially ambiguous local assessments of ABMR based on conventional features (histology, C4d staining, and DSA), a single pathologist in Edmonton read all the reports to ensure that the diagnoses recorded in the Scientific Data Management System represented the opinion of the local center as stated in the pathology report. For comparison with the BFC403 reference set, and without knowledge of the ABMR scores, these diagnoses were then assigned into categories as previously defined.[20]

Positive correlative findings between ABMR and conventional features (histology, C4d staining, and DSA) were similarly observed for the INT300 set. In particular, the ABMR score of greater than 0.2 correlated with ABMR lesions, as well as with IF/TA and arteriolar hyalinosis, which are Banff consensus diagnostic features of ABMR.[6] The ABMR score was also higher in biopsies from DSA+ patients at the time of biopsy compared with those who were DSA− or without HLA antibody. Overall, the agreement between the 2 diagnostic methods was similar to that in the BFC403 reference set with an accuracy of approximately 85% in both.[10]

Although the ABMR score in C4d− ABMR was similar to C4d+ ABMR, confirming longstanding suspicions of C4d staining accuracy, the authors point out that positive correlations between the ABMR score and reference points such as lesion grades, DSA, and survival, are reassuring, and ultimately the ABMR score was more strongly associated with graft failure than conventional assessment (**Fig. 3**). The ABMR score was first compared with the local conventional assessment of ABMR for prediction of 3-year graft survival in patients with late biopsies (>1 year posttransplant). Although both diagnostic methods were associated with prediction of graft loss on univariable analysis, only the ABMR score was significantly associated with graft loss in the INT300 set when multivariable analyses were applied.[10] **Fig. 3** illustrates that when the ABMR score was positive (S+), graft loss was rapid in the first year posttransplant, regardless of the local assessment (S+C+ and S + C−). Even more striking was that in cases more than 3 years postbiopsy, where ABMR was not diagnosed locally (C−) but received an ABMR (S+) score, there was significantly lower graft survival than in cases that were diagnosed locally but did not receive an ABMR score greater than 0.2 (S−C+) ($P = .003$ by log-rank test). In summary, when there was a disagreement between the 2 diagnoses, only the ABMR score was associated with early progression to failure.

The results from the INTERCOM study also documented the uncertainty in conventional assessment previously observed in the BFC403 reference set. In 41% of the INT300 biopsies, where ABMR features were noted by pathologists, their recorded diagnoses did not conclude ABMR. Instead, transplant glomerulopathy was often chosen as the diagnosis, which is not equivalent to ABMR.[28] The ABMR score was highly correlative with ABMR histologic lesions and DSA, but not with T-cell–mediated rejection lesions. In a follow-up review article, this group further elaborates on these not unexpected discrepancies.[9] The authors point out that there is not a singular phenotype of ABMR, and this also can change over time posttransplant, complicating the diagnosis.[26,29] Possible sources for these discrepancies are suggested to be various combinations of false-positive histology or DSA, or alternatively, false-negative molecular

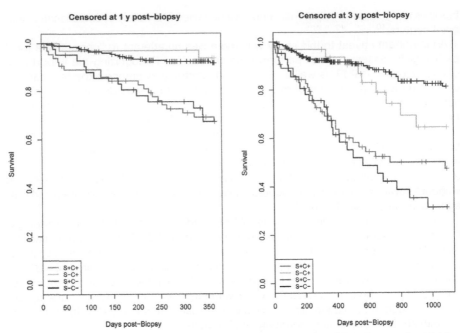

Fig. 3. Kaplan–Meier graft survival curves. Based on one random biopsy per patient in the patients receiving late (>1-year posttransplantation) biopsies in the INT300. The ABMR score is dichotomized into S+ (>0.2) and S− (≤0.2), as is the conventional assessment of ABMR/mixed as C+ and C− by the local center. (*Data from* Halloran PF, Pereira AB, Chang J, et al. Potential impact of microarray diagnosis of T cell-mediated rejection in kidney transplants: the INTERCOM study. Am J Transplant 2013;13(9):2352–63.)

scores as well as genuine heterogeneity in kidney disease, which is accepted in lesion scoring and most likely an intrinsic part of ABMR phenotypes based on antibody specificity, disease activity, and disease duration.

The most recent large-scale clinical study by this group, using the MMDx molecular diagnostic system, was an extension of the INTERCOM trial, named INTERCOMEX, which details the prospective trial undertaken to assess the feasibility of real-time central molecular assessment of kidney transplant biopsy samples from 10 North American or European centers. For this study, 519 biopsies were obtained 1 day to 34 years posttransplantation, and sent overnight to the central laboratory to be processed immediately, or stored at −20°C. Diagnoses were assigned based only on the ABMR score generated from the MMDx system, blinded to histology or HLA antibody status, and signed out by one observer. The premise for this undertaking of requiring a centralized laboratory was based on the assumption that microarrays, if processed in multiple laboratories, would yield enough variation in measurements as to make the classifiers unreliable. The INTERCOMEX study used a comparator group that combined the BFC403 reference set with the INT300 biopsies,[10,18] termed "Population 703."[5] This study also described new classifiers that were derived from previous rejection diagnoses.[15] Results again supported earlier correlative findings between ABMR score and histologic diagnosis of ABMR, with the overall accuracy assessments for prediction of a histologic diagnosis of rejection being as follows: Sensitivity 78%, Specificity 74%, PPV 90%, NPV 54%, and a balanced accuracy of 76%.

The promise of the utility of this molecular diagnostic tool was evident from the feedback received for 451 of the INTERCOMEX biopsy samples. The clinical feedback indicated that clinicians agreed with MMDx more often than with their local biopsy assessment and stated that MMDx would give them more confidence in their clinical management decisions. Ultimately, the report accuracy of 76% to 77% for a sign-out diagnosis of rejection was significant because the researchers had also created a classification tree for predicting the pathologists' diagnoses, to establish an automated sign-out in the absence of an individual experts' interpretation. For this, they were able to successfully provide an automated prediction of the pathologists' sign-outs with 90% accuracy.

A

Pure Molecular Interpretation (Results Summary)

Very active ABMR, with ptc, g, and cg molecular features. No TCMR. Extensive inflammation. Moderate AKI and atrophy-fibrosis.	Percent cortex[a]
	79%

Result Details

Biopsy Rejection and Injury Scores

	Classifier / Gene Sets	Biopsy Score	Range of Values[b]	Upper Limit of Normal[c]	Interpretation
Injury Scores	Global Disturbance Score	2.63	−3.8 − 5.8	0.03	Moderate
	Acute Kidney Injury (AKI) Score	0.65	−0.6 − 1.6	0.39	Mild
	Atrophy-Fibrosis Score	0.47	0 − 1	0.76	Mild
Rejection Scores	Rejection Score	0.95	0 − 1	0.30	Severe
	T Cell-Mediated Rejection (TCMR) Score	0.02	0 − 1	0.10	Normal
	Antibody-Mediated Rejection (ABMR) Score	0.96	0 − 1	0.20	Severe

Archetypal Analysis (please see Archetypal Analysis Description on Page 2 for details)

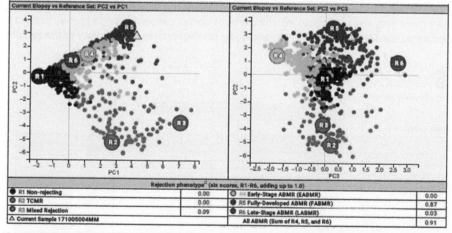

Rejection phenotype[d] (six scores, R1-R6, adding up to 1.0)			
● R1 Non-rejecting	0.00	○ Early-Stage ABMR (EABMR)	0.00
● R2 TCMR	0.00	● R5 Fully-Developed ABMR (FABMR)	0.87
● R3 Mixed Rejection	0.09	● R6 Late-Stage ABMR (LABMR)	0.03
△ Current Sample 171005004MM		All ABMR (Sum of R4, R5, and R6)	0.91

Fig. 4. MMDx report for a sample with fully developed ABMR. (*A*) The results are summarized in the Pure Molecular Interpretation section. The main injury and rejection classifiers are shown along with their interpretations. Archetypal analysis is used to define a set of pure rejection phenotypes or archetypes (nonrejection, TCMR, stages of ABMR, and mixed) within the reference biopsy data set. A visualization of the same data set, produced by principal component analysis, is shown. The axes represent molecular continua: PC1 is nonrejection to rejection (*left to right*); PC2 is ABMR to TCMR (*top to bottom*); and PC3 is early to late-stage ABMR (*left to right*). PC3 can be thought of as the view down the x axis of the PC2 versus PC1 figure. Scores for the probability of each archetype for the current biopsy are given below the plots. (*B*) Survival percentages are then given as well as results on other classifiers including those based on histologic lesions. Nearest neighbor analysis provides results for the histologic diagnoses of the 50 nearest molecular neighbors. [a] Percent cortex is a quality control measure. [b] The 2.5th to 97.5th percentiles in the entire Reference Set. [c] 90th percentile in relevant Reference Set biopsies. [d] Scores from archetypal analysis.

RESULTS PROVIDED BY MOLECULAR MICROSCOPE TESTING

The kidney biopsy microarray data are used to produce the MMDx test report, which incorporates all of the aforementioned analysis and provides clinicians with scores for their specific biopsy. Each new biopsy's molecular profile is compared with those in the large reference set of fully annotated biopsies and a diagnosis is made.[15] For the TCMR, ABMR, and all rejection classifiers, a score between 0.0 and 1.0 is given that indicates the probability of the respective conventional diagnosis.[19,20,30] In addition, an interpretation of each score as minimal, mild, moderate, or severe (for the injury scores) and normal, mild, moderate, or severe (for the rejection scores) is given (**Fig. 4**A). Biopsy scores that are based on histologic lesions are also provided (**Fig. 4**B). The diagnostic interpretation is therefore based on the integration of several estimates provided on the report. Chief among these are the rejection, ABMR, and TCMR scores, as well as the 6 rejection phenotype scores (R1 nonrejecting, R2 TCMR, R3 mixed rejection, R4 early-stage ABMR, R5 fully developed ABMR, R6 late-stage ABMR). Injury is also assessed, primarily using the global disturbance, AKI, and atrophy-disturbance scores. Related to both of these (rejection and injury) is the ah-probability: an indicator of possible nonadherence. A visualization of the reference biopsy data, produced by principal components analysis, is given with the current biopsy's scores for the probability of each archetype (see **Fig. 4**A).

A survival percentage is also given for biopsies in the proprietary reference set that have scores similar to that of the tested biopsy (see **Fig. 4**B).[21] An advantage of the MMDx system, unlike conventional pathology, is that it can read medulla. However, some classifiers may require additional interpretation if the percentage of medulla in a sample is very high.[31] Therefore, the percent cortex present in each biopsy is calculated using the MMDx software and provided on the reports. A summary of the results

B

Survival Compared to Reference Set

Survival in patients with similar biopsies in the Reference Set			
1 Year	71%	3 Year	55%

Additional Biopsy Scores

	Classifier / Gene Sets	Biopsy Score	Range of Values[c]	Upper Limit of Normal[f]	Interpretation
TCMR Related	TCMR-1	0.02	0 – 1	0.10	Normal
	TCMR-2	0.02	0 – 1	0.10	Normal
	Mean of 2 TCMR Classifiers	0.02	0 – 1	0.10	Normal
Rejection Related	Rejection	0.95	0 – 1	0.30	Severe
Injury-Scarring Related	AKI Score	0.65	−0.6 – 1.5	0.39	Mild
	Atrophy-Fibrosis Score	0.47	0 – 1	0.75	Mild
ABMR Related	ABMR-1	0.96	0 – 1	0.20	Severe
	ABMR-2	0.91	0 – 1	0.20	Severe
	ABMR-3	0.97	0 – 1	0.20	Severe
	Mean of 3 ABMR Classifiers	0.95	0 – 1	0.20	Severe
Classifiers based on Histologic Lesions	Glomerulitie (g) >0 probability	0.85	0 – 1	0.34	Severe
	Transplant Glomerulopathy (cg) >0 Probability	0.94	0 – 1	0.24	Severe
	Peritubular capillaritis (ptc) >0	0.87	0 – 1	0.26	Severe
	DSA-positive probability	0.83	0 – 1	0.48	Severe
	Interstitial inflammation (i) >1 probability	0.38	0 – 1	0.08	Moderate
	Tubulitis (t) >1 probability	0.12	0 – 1	0.12	Normal
	Tubular atrophy (ct) >1 probability	0.33	0 – 1	0.87	Normal
	Arteriolar hyalinosis (ah) >0 probability	0.70	0 – 1	0.91	Normal

For Classifiers:
TCMR-1 TCMR vs everything else.
ABMR-1 ABMR vs everything else.
ABMR-3 ABMR vs everything else, with Mixed/TG/ABMR suspicious withheld.

TCMR-2 TCMR vs everything else, with BK/Borderline/Mixed withheld.
ABMR-2 ABMR vs everything else, with TG/ABMR suspicious withheld.

Nearest Neighbor Analysis

Rank order of the most common histologic diagnoses in the 50 nearest molecular neighbors.	
ABMR	70%
NOMOA	8%
Mixed	8%
TG	4%
GN	4%

Mean molecular scores in the 50 nearest molecular neighbors.	
ABMR	0.9
Rej	0.88
Acute Kidney Injury	0.53
Atrophy-Fibrosis	0.52
TCMR	0.03

Fig. 4. (*continued*).

is written by an experienced observer, making note of whether rejection is present, the level of inflammation present, and the levels of AKI or atrophy-fibrosis present (see **Fig. 4**A). The comprehensive analysis of the biopsy and the resulting report provides the clinician with a complete assessment of the graft status, which can be used alongside or in place of conventional assessment.

SUMMARY

The authors thus concluded that evidence from these cumulative studies supports the implementation of a central molecular interpretation test that can offer an objective "second opinion," adding another dimension to the pathologists' local histology findings that could have value when faced with uncertainty in histology diagnoses. They propose that one strength of the molecular system is that many classifiers can be applied, differing in their training algorithms; analogous to asking many pathologists to read a single biopsy. As the MMDx system evolves, many separate classifiers for TCMR or for ABMR can be developed, such that the end result will be a consensus among many independent estimates.[9] ATAGC has continued their efforts to this effect and has recently shown that generating a probability estimate using regression equations based on lesion scores and DSA assessments maximizes the diagnostic accuracy, and can estimate probability for ABMR when DSA is unknown or undetectable.[32]

REFERENCES

1. Wekerle T, Segev D, Lechler R, et al. Strategies for long-term preservation of kidney graft function. Lancet 2017;389(10084):2152–62.
2. Hart A, Smith JM, Skeans MA, et al. OPTN/SRTR 2016 annual data report: kidney. Am J Transplant 2018;18(Suppl 1):18–113.
3. Einecke G, Sis B, Reeve J, et al. Antibody-mediated microcirculation injury is the major cause of late kidney transplant failure. Am J Transplant 2009;9(11): 2520–31.
4. Kurian SM, Williams AN, Gelbart T, et al. Molecular classifiers for acute kidney transplant rejection in peripheral blood by whole genome gene expression profiling. Am J Transplant 2014;14(5):1164–72.
5. Halloran PF, Chang J, Famulski K, et al. Disappearance of T cell-mediated rejection despite continued antibody-mediated rejection in late kidney transplant recipients. J Am Soc Nephrol 2015;26(7):1711–20.
6. Solez K, Colvin RB, Racusen LC, et al. Banff 07 classification of renal allograft pathology: updates and future directions. Am J Transplant 2008;8(4):753–60.
7. Loupy A, Hill GS, Suberbielle C, et al. Significance of C4d Banff scores in early protocol biopsies of kidney transplant recipients with preformed donor-specific antibodies (DSA). Am J Transplant 2011;11(1):56–65.
8. Haas M, Sis B, Racusen LC, et al. Banff 2013 meeting report: inclusion of c4d-negative antibody-mediated rejection and antibody-associated arterial lesions. Am J Transplant 2014;14(2):272–83.
9. Halloran PF, Famulski KS, Reeve J. Molecular assessment of disease states in kidney transplant biopsy samples. Nat Rev Nephrol 2016;12(9):534–48.
10. Halloran PF, Pereira AB, Chang J, et al. Microarray diagnosis of antibody-mediated rejection in kidney transplant biopsies: an international prospective study (INTERCOM). Am J Transplant 2013;13(11):2865–74.

11. de Freitas DG, Sellarés J, Mengel M, et al. The nature of biopsies with "borderline rejection" and prospects for eliminating this category. Am J Transplant 2012; 12(1):191–201.

12. Hirt-Minkowski P, De Serres SA, Ho J. Developing renal allograft surveillance strategies—urinary biomarkers of cellular rejection. Can J Kidney Health Dis 2015;2:28.

13. Roedder S, Sigdel T, Salomonis N, et al. The kSORT assay to detect renal transplant patients at high risk for acute rejection: results of the multicenter AART study. PLoS Med 2014;11(11):e1001759.

14. Bloom RD, Bromberg JS, Poggio ED, et al. Cell-free DNA and active rejection in kidney allografts. J Am Soc Nephrol 2017;28(7):2221–32.

15. Halloran PF, Reeve J, Akalin E, et al. Real time central assessment of kidney transplant indication biopsies by microarrays: the INTERCOMEX study. Am J Transplant 2017;17(11):2851–62.

16. Halloran PF, de Freitas DG, Einecke G, et al. The molecular phenotype of kidney transplants. Am J Transplant 2010;10(10):2215–22.

17. Halloran PF, Famulski K, Reeve J. The molecular phenotypes of rejection in kidney transplant biopsies. Curr Opin Organ Transplant 2015;20(3):359–67.

18. Halloran PF, Pereira AB, Chang J, et al. Potential impact of microarray diagnosis of T cell-mediated rejection in kidney transplants: the INTERCOM study. Am J Transplant 2013;13(9):2352–63.

19. Reeve J, Sellarés J, Mengel M, et al. Molecular diagnosis of T cell-mediated rejection in human kidney transplant biopsies. Am J Transplant 2013;13(3):645–55.

20. Sellarés J, Reeve J, Loupy A, et al. Molecular diagnosis of antibody-mediated rejection in human kidney transplants. Am J Transplant 2013;13(4):971–83.

21. Einecke G, Reeve J, Sis B, et al. A molecular classifier for predicting future graft loss in late kidney transplant biopsies. J Clin Invest 2010;120(6):1862–72.

22. Famulski KS, de Freitas DG, Kreepala C, et al. Molecular phenotypes of acute kidney injury in kidney transplants. J Am Soc Nephrol 2012;23(5):948–58.

23. Famulski KS, Reeve J, de Freitas DG, et al. Kidney transplants with progressing chronic diseases express high levels of acute kidney injury transcripts. Am J Transplant 2013;13(3):634–44.

24. Venner JM, Famulski KS, Reeve J, et al. Relationships among injury, fibrosis, and time in human kidney transplants. JCI Insight 2016;1(1):e85323.

25. Reeve J. Core PBTs gene list. 2017. Available at: https://www.ualberta.ca/medicine/institutes-centres-groups/atagc/research/gene-lists. Accessed April 2, 2018.

26. Halloran PF, Merino Lopez M, Barreto Pereira A. Identifying subphenotypes of antibody-mediated rejection in kidney transplants. Am J Transplant 2016;16(3):908–20.

27. Sis B, Mengel M, Haas M, et al. Banff '09 meeting report: antibody mediated graft deterioration and implementation of Banff working groups. Am J Transplant 2010;10(3):464–71.

28. Baid-Agrawal S, Farris AB, Pascual M, et al. Overlapping pathways to transplant glomerulopathy: chronic humoral rejection, hepatitis C infection, and thrombotic microangiopathy. Kidney Int 2011;80(8):879–85.

29. Sellarés J, de Freitas DG, Mengel M, et al. Understanding the causes of kidney transplant failure: the dominant role of antibody-mediated rejection and nonadherence. Am J Transplant 2012;12(2):388–99.

30. Reeve J, Einecke G, Mengel M, et al. Diagnosing rejection in renal transplants: a comparison of molecular- and histopathology-based approaches. Am J Transplant 2009;9(8):1802–10.

31. Madill-Thomsen KS, Wiggins RC, Eskandary F, et al. The effect of cortex/medulla proportions on molecular diagnoses in kidney transplant biopsies: rejection and injury can be assessed in medulla. Am J Transplant 2017;17(8):2117–28.
32. Halloran PF, Famulski KS, Chang J. A probabilistic approach to histologic diagnosis of antibody-mediated rejection in kidney transplant biopsies. Am J Transplant 2017;17(1):129–39.

Diversity of Killer Cell Immunoglobulin-Like Receptors and Disease

Raja Rajalingam, PhD

KEYWORDS

- Natural killer (NK) cells • Killer cell immunoglobulin-like receptors (KIR)
- Human leukocyte antigen (HLA) • Innate immunity
- Inhibitory and activating receptors • KIR polymorphism and diversity
- Genetic association with disease • Hematopoietic stem cell transplantation (HST)

KEY POINTS

- Natural killer (NK) cells are the third population of lymphocytes that involve in the innate immunity controlling infections and malignancies. NK cells also contribute to adaptive immune responses.
- NK cells use a variety of germline-encoded cell surface receptors to discriminate target cells from the healthy cells. Killer cell immunoglobulin-like receptors (KIR) are the key receptors for human NK cells. KIR binds certain conserved motives of the polymorphic human leukocyte antigen (HLA) class molecules.
- During the development, KIRs bind cognate HLA class I molecules, which trigger NK cell maturation process (termed licensing or education). Licensing enables NK cells to survey, recognize, and kill stressed target cells that lost HLA class I molecules as a consequence of viral infection and tumor transformation.
- Genes encoding KIRs and HLA class I ligands are located on different chromosomes, and both feature extraordinary diversity in the number and type of genes. The independent segregation of unlinked KIR and HLA gene families produce exceptional diversity in the number and type of KIR-HLA gene combinations inherited in individuals.
- KIR-HLA genetic variation affects KIR repertoire of NK cell clones, NK cell maturation, and thus influence the capability to deliver signals, which may affect NK cell response on infections, tumor transformation, autoimmune diseases, and allogeneic transplantation.

NATURAL KILLER CELL IMMUNITY

Natural killer (NK) cells are bone marrow–derived large granular lymphocytes defined by CD3^{neg}CD56^{pos} and represent 5% to 25% of peripheral blood mononuclear cell

Disclosure: The author has nothing to disclose.
Department of Surgery, Immunogenetics and Transplantation Laboratory, University of California San Francisco, 3333 California Street, Suite 150, San Francisco, CA 94118, USA
E-mail address: Rajalingam.Raja@ucsf.edu

Clin Lab Med 38 (2018) 637–653
https://doi.org/10.1016/j.cll.2018.08.001
0272-2712/18/© 2018 Elsevier Inc. All rights reserved.

labmed.theclinics.com

fraction of the healthy humans. NK cells were originally described as innate lympho-cytes capable of mounting early immune responses by lysing target cells via direct cytotoxicity in an antigen-independent manner quickly, without a "priming" period as required for T cells.[1] But now, NK cells are recognized to express a complex reper-toire of activating and inhibitory receptors that is calibrated to ensure self-tolerance while exerting early assaults against viral infection[2] and tumor transformation.[3] Furthermore, NK cells can mount antigen-specific immunologic memory, a hallmark attribute of adaptive immunity.[4] In addition to cytolysis, the NK cells also produce a wide range of both proinflammatory and immunosuppressive cytokines, as well as many chemokines that contribute to the outcome of adaptive immune responses.[5]

NK cells share several features with cytotoxic T lymphocytes (CTL) in development, morphology, cell-surface phenotypes, and effector functions but differ substantially in their cell surface receptors used to recognize infected/transformed target cells.[6] The CTL binds class I human leukocyte antigen (HLA) and its bound peptide complex expressed on target cells through specific T-cell receptors, which trigger cytolysis of infected target cells. Many viruses have evolved strategies to evade the CTL response by specifically downregulating class I HLA in the infected cell, which allows the virus to prevent its host cell from presenting viral-derived peptides to CTLs. The aberrant levels of class I expression due to viral infections, neoplastic transformations, or other forms of stress permit NK cells to eliminate these unhealthy target cells (**Fig. 1**). NK cells use their inhibitory receptors to detect the absence of self-HLA

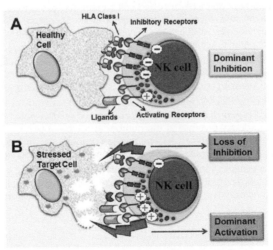

Fig. 1. Dynamic regulation of NK cell response against healthy and unhealthy stressed target cells. NK cells express both inhibitory and activating receptors, and the net signal in-tegrated from these inhibitory and activating receptors determines the effector function of NK cells. Inhibitory receptors recognize self-HLA class I molecules and trigger signals that stop the natural lytic function of NK cells. By expressing normal levels of HLA-A, -B, and -C molecules, the healthy cells become resistant to NK surveillance (A). Downregulation of HLA class I expression due to tumor transformation or viral infection relieves the inhibi-tory influence on NK cells (B), permitting NK cells to lyse these unhealthy target cells, a phe-nomenon first described as the "missing-self" hypothesis. On transformation or infection, the unhealthy cells express ligands for activating receptors, which could be either "induced-self" (major histocompatibility complex class I-like chains A and B, unique long binding protein), "altered-self" (HLA-class I loaded with foreign peptide), and/or "non-self" (pathogen encoded molecules). On recognizing these ligands, the activating receptors trigger signals that augment NK cell lysis of unhealthy targets.

molecules on potential target cells—a recognition strategy that is known as the detection of "missing-self" hypothesis.[7,8] Abundant expression of 4 distinct HLA class I molecules (HLA-A, -B, -C, and -E) on normal healthy cells provide ligands for a variety of inhibitory receptors of NK cells and consequently are resistant to NK cell attack. In addition to the "missing-self" mechanism, the activation receptors that can directly recognize stress-induced ligands associated with infection and tumor transformation, might also contribute to NK cell attack.[9] The ligands identified for activating receptors are either "induced-self" (such as major histocompatibility complex [MHC] class I-like chains A and B and unique long binding proteins), "altered-self" (HLA class I molecules loaded with foreign peptide), or pathogen-encoded "non-self" molecules associated with infection and tumor transformation. Therefore, the net signal integrated from the inhibitory and activating receptors determines the effector function of NK cells.[9]

KILLER CELL IMMUNOGLOBULIN-LIKE RECEPTORS

NK cells have a highly specific and sophisticated target cell recognition receptor system arbitrated by the integration of signals triggered by a multitude of inhibitory and activating receptors.[10,11] Unlike T-cell receptor that is generated by somatic gene rearrangements, NK cells use a wide array of conventional germline-encoded receptor repertoire.[9,12] Human NK cells express distinct families of receptors, including (1) killer cell immunoglobulin-like receptors (KIR), (2) killer cell lectin-like receptors, (3) leukocyte immunoglobulin-like receptors (LILR), and (4) natural cytotoxicity receptors.[9,12–14]

The KIRs are considered to be the key receptors that control the development and function of human NK cells.[12,15–18] Fourteen KIRs triggering either inhibition (3DL1-3, 2DL1-3, 2DL5) or activation (3DS1, 2DS1-5), or both (2DL4) have been identified in humans (**Fig. 2**).[19,20] KIRs possess 2 or 3 extracellular immunoglobulin (Ig)-like domains involved in ligand binding and either a long or a short cytoplasmic tail associated with signaling function. KIRs are named on the basis of their number of Ig domains and type of cytoplasmic tail.[21] The first digit following the KIR acronym corresponds to the number of Ig-like domains in the molecule and the "D" denotes "domain." The "D" is followed by either an "L" indicating a "Long" cytoplasmic tail, an "S" indicating a "Short" cytoplasmic tail, or a "P" for pseudogenes (2DP1 and 3DP1). The final digit indicates the number of the gene encoding a protein with this structure. Thus KIR2DL1, KIR2DL2, and KIR2DL3 all encode receptors having 2 extracellular Ig-like domains and long cytoplasmic tails, whereas KIR3DS1 encodes a receptor having 3 extracellular Ig-like domains and a short cytoplasmic tail. Long tails are characteristic of the inhibitory forms and contain 1 or 2 copies of immunoreceptor tyrosine-based inhibition motifs (ITIMs) that become phosphorylated on interaction with specific HLA class I ligand and recruit Src homology region 2 domain containing phosphatase 1 and 2 that switch off NK cell responses. The short-tailed activating KIRs lack ITIMs, whereas they are characterized by a positively charged amino acid residue in the transmembrane region that allows the interaction with the DAP-12 (DNAX activation protein of 12 kDa). The DAP12 adapter chain contains immunoreceptor tyrosine-based activation motifs, which trigger activating signals on the short-tailed KIR bound to a relevant ligand.

EXTRAORDINARY DIVERSITY OF KILLER CELL IMMUNOGLOBULIN-LIKE RECEPTOR SYSTEM

KIR system differs from other types of NK cell receptors by its substantial diversity, which is contributed by multiple factors, such as individual-specific KIR gene content, nucleotide sequence polymorphism of each KIR gene, stochastic and variegated

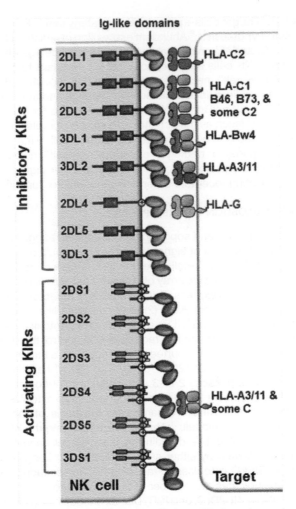

Fig. 2. KIRs and HLA class I ligands. Fourteen distinct KIRs have been characterized in humans, comprising either 2 or 3 (2-domains [2D] or 3D) extracellular Ig-like domains and either a long (*L*) or short (*S*) cytoplasmic tail. Six KIRs are activating types and the remaining KIRs are inhibitory types. The cytoplasmic tails of the inhibitory KIRs carry immunoreceptor tyrosine-based inhibition motif (ITIM) (shown as *blue boxes*) that trigger inhibitory signals on binding to distinct HLA class I ligands. The short-tailed activating KIRs lack ITIM but carry a positively charged amino acid residue in the transmembrane region (shown by *yellow circle* with + mark) that allows the interaction with an adapter chain DAP12. The DAP12 contains immunoreceptor tyrosine-based activation motifs (shown as *red boxes*), which trigger activating signals on the short-tailed KIR bound to a relevant ligand. The ligands for most activating KIRs are unknown.

expression of KIR repertoires on individual NK cell clones, and functional threshold acquirement during NK cell development by interacting with individual-specific cognate HLA class I ligands.

KIRs are encoded by a family of tightly clustered homologous genes on the leukocyte receptor complex that spans a region of about 150 kb on chromosome 19q13.4.[19,20] The number and type of KIR genes vary substantially between haplotypes (**Fig. 3**). More than 30 distinct KIR haplotypes with distinct gene content have been characterized to date by sequencing genomic clones and haplotype segregation analysis in families. On the basis of gene content, KIR haplotypes are broadly classified into 2 groups.[22] Group A haplotypes have a fixed gene content (KIR3DL3-2DL3-2DP1-2DL1-3DP1-2DL4-3DL1-2DS4-3DL2) that encode 4 inhibitory KIRs, 2DL1, 2DL3, 3DL1, and 3DL2, specific for 4 major HLA class I ligands, C2, C1, Bw4, and A3/A11 respectively, and an activating KIR 2DS4, which is weakly specific for some HLA-C allotypes (C1 or C2 epitope), as well as the HLA-A3/11 epitope. In contrast, group B haplotypes are variable both in numbers and combinations of KIR genes and comprise several genes (2DL2, 2DL5, 2DS1, 2DS2, 2DS3, 2DS5, 3DS1) that are not part of the A haplotype. Moreover, B haplotypes possess KIRs that have no or decreased binding to HLA class I ligands, such as KIR2DS2, KIR2DS3, and KIR2DS5. Although group A haplotypes contain only KIR2DS4 as an activating gene, group B haplotypes contain up to 5 activating KIRs—KIR2DS1, 2DS2, 2DS3, 2DS5, and 3DS1. The gene content varies dramatically between group-B haplotypes. Inheritance of paternal and maternal haplotypes comprising different KIR gene content haplotypes (A + A, A + B, or B + B) generates extraordinary diversity between humans.

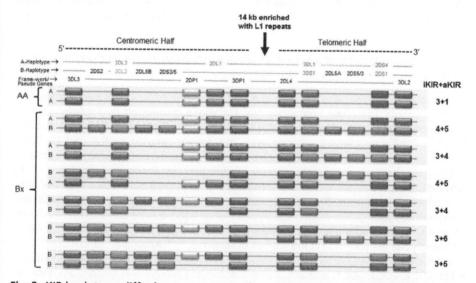

Fig. 3. KIR haplotypes differ by gene content. The number and type of KIR genes vary substantially between haplotypes. On the basis of gene content, KIR haplotypes are broadly classified into 2 groups. Group A haplotypes have a fixed gene content (KIR3DL3-2DL3-2DP1-2DL1-3DP1-2DL4-3DL1-2DS4-3DL2). In contrast, group B haplotypes are variable both in numbers and combinations of KIR genes and comprising several genes (2DL2, 2DL5, 2DS1, 2DS2, 2DS3, 2DS5, 3DS1) that are not part of the A haplotype. Although group A haplotypes contain only KIR2DS4 as an activating gene, group B haplotypes contain up to 5 activating KIRs—KIR2DS1, 2DS2, 2DS3, 2DS5, and 3DS1. A stretch of 14 kb enriched with L1 repeats upstream of KIR2DL4 divides the KIR haplotype into 2 halves. The centromeric half is delimited by 3DL3 and 3DP1, whereas the telomeric half is delimited by 2DL4 and 3DL2. Multiple reciprocal meiotic recombination events between 3DP1 and 2DL4 shuffle the centromeric and telomeric motifs and thus diversify gene content KIR haplotypes across individuals and populations. Inheritance of paternal and maternal haplotypes comprising different KIR gene content haplotypes (A + A, A + B, or B + B) generates extraordinary inhibitory (iKIR) and activating KIR (aKIR) gene content diversity between humans.

Only 4 KIR genes (3DL3, 3DP1, 2DL4, and 3DL2) present on all haplotypes are referred to as "framework" genes. KIR3DL3 and 3DL2 mark the centeromeric and telomeric boundaries of the KIR gene complex respectively, whereas 3DP1 and 2DL4 are located in the middle of the KIR gene complex. KIR3DP1 and 2DL4 genes are separated by a 14 kb sequence enriched with L1 repeats, whereas the distance between other KIR genes is only a 2 kb homogeneous sequence. The 14 kb DNA sequence between 3DP1 and 2DL4 divides the KIR haplotypes into 2 halves.[19] KIR3DL3 at the 5′-end and 3DP1 at the 3′-end mark the centromeric half, whereas 2DL4 at the 5′-end and 3DL2 at the 3′-end mark the telomeric half. In contrast, the existence of the other 12 KIR genes is considerably variable. The inhibitory receptors KIR2DL2 and 2DL3 segregate as alleles of a single locus at the centromeric half. Similarly, the inhibitory KIR3DL1 and activating KIR3DS1 behave as alleles of the same locus at the telomeric half. Almost all haplotypes contain these 2 loci, such that virtually everyone has either 2DL2 or 2DL3 and 3DL1 or 3DS1 within their KIR genome. KIR2DL1, 2DL2, 2DL3, and 2DS2 are specific to the centromeric half, whereas KIR3DL1, 3DS1, 2DS1, and 2DS4 are specific to the telomeric half. Three KIR genes, 2DL5, 2DS3, and 2DS5, are found in both centromeric and telomeric locations.[23,24] For genes within each half there is significant linkage disequilibrium but much less for genes in the 2 different halves.[25–28] Multiple reciprocal recombination events at the center of the KIR complex, between 3DP1 and 2DL4, presumably diversify gene content for KIR haplotypes across individuals and populations.[27,29]

POPULATION DIVERSITY IN KILLER CELL IMMUNOGLOBULIN-LIKE RECEPTOR GENE CONTENT

All human populations have both group A and B haplotypes, but their frequencies vary considerably.[30] The Allele Frequency Net Database developed by Professor Derek Middleton compiles the frequency of KIR genes and genotypes in different populations[31] (http://www.allelefrequencies.net/). Individuals carrying both A and B haplotypes are more common in Caucasians and Africans, and therefore A and B haplotypes are approximately equally distributed in these populations.[22,27] In contrast, the prevalence of inhibitory haplotypes (group-A) dominates over the activating haplotypes (group-B) in one population and vice versa in others. Individuals carrying homozygous group-A KIR haplotypes (AA genotypes) are common in Northeast Asians (Chinese, Japanese, and Koreans).[32–34] Conversely, individuals carrying AB or BB genotypes are common in the natives of America,[35,36] Australia,[37] and India.[30,38,39] The NK cells from AA homozygous individuals can express a maximum of 4 inhibitory KIRs (2DL1, 2DL3, 3DL1, and 3DL2) and 1 activating KIR (2DS4). In contrast, individuals carrying AB or BB genotypes can express a maximum of 6 inhibitory KIRs (2DL1-3, 2DL5, 3DL1, and 3DL2) and 2 to 6 activating KIRs (3DS1, 2DS1-5). NK cells of group-B haplotype carriers express more activating KIRs and respond more vigorously to pathogens. These data suggest that the aboriginal populations of India, Australia, and America acquired activating KIR genes to survive the environmental challenges during their extensive prehistoric migrations from Africa.[30]

ALLELIC DIVERSITY OF KILLER CELL IMMUNOGLOBULIN-LIKE RECEPTOR GENES

In addition to haplotypic diversity, each KIR gene exhibits considerable sequence polymorphism.[25,40] Inhibitory KIRs are more polymorphic than the activating KIRs. The highest allelic polymorphisms are reported for 3DL1, 3DL2, and 3DL3 loci, which is probably due to the subjective sequencing analyses of large cohorts by certain laboratories that focus on these loci.[40–43] The framework genes KIR3DL2 and 3DL3 are relatively more polymorphic, whereas the activating KIR genes are generally conserved. The functional consequence of sequence polymorphism has been studied in great detail for the KIR3DL1 locus. The amino acid substitutions that distinguish allelic diversity of 3DL1 are enriched in polymorphic HLA-Bw4 ligand binding Ig-like domains compared with the cytoplasmic tail region, and such diversity seems to be the result of natural selection.[40] The sequence polymorphisms of KIR3DL1, KIR2DL1, and KIR2DL2/3 are shown to influence their expression, ligand binding, and cytolytic and cytokine secretion functions.[41,44–52] Some KIR sequences are null alleles that carry either a premature stop codon or one or more nucleotide substitution/deletion/insertions that alter the reading frame of protein synthesis, which affect their cell surface expression. The synergistic combination of allelic polymorphism and variable gene content individualize KIR genotypes to an extent where unrelated individuals almost always have different KIR types.[25] This level of diversity likely reflects a strong pressure from pathogens on the human NK cell response.

LIGANDS FOR KILLER CELL IMMUNOGLOBULIN-LIKE RECEPTORS

KIRs recognize specific motifs of HLA class I molecules, which are the products of highly polymorphic genes of the MHC that comprises about 3.6 Mb DNA on the short arm of chromosome 6 (6p21.3).[53,54] The human MHC contains 6 functional HLA class I genes. Of these, the polymorphic HLA-A, HLA-B, and HLA-C genes encode classical class I molecules, whereas conserved HLA-E, HLA-F, and HLA-G genes encode nonclassical class I molecules. Except HLA-F, all class I molecules are known to interact with NK cell receptors. Each HLA-A, HLA-B, or HLA-C allotype either carries 1 of the 4 epitopes recognized by KIR, A3/11, Bw4, C1, or C2 or has none of these epitopes and does not function as a KIR ligand. No HLA-A, HLA-B, or HLA-C allotype carries more than 1 of the 4 epitopes, thus they are mutually exclusive.

All known alleles of HLA-C have either asparagine (HLA-C*01, C*03, C*07, C*08, C*12, C*14, and C*16—termed C1 epitope) or lysine (HLA-C*02, C*04, C*05, C*06, C*15, C*17, and C*18—termed C2 epitope) at position 80 located in the F-pocket of the peptide-binding groove, and these dimorphic epitopes are recognized by different isoforms of KIR2D.[55–58] Epitopes C1 and C2 are recognized by the inhibitory KIR2DL2/3 and KIR2DL1 receptors, respectively (see **Fig. 2**). The inhibitory signals triggered by the KIR2DL2/3+HLA-C1 interaction are relatively weak as compared with those triggered by the KIR2DL1+HLA-C2 interaction.[45] KIR3DL1 binds to the Bw4 epitope, defined by amino acid residues 77 to 83 in the α1 domain,[59–61] which is present on approximately 40% of the HLA-B allotypes (B13, B27, B37, B38, B44, B47, B49, B51, B52, B53, B57, B58, B59, B63, B77) and 17% of HLA-A allotypes (HLA-A23, 24, 25, and 32). Around 50% of HLA haplotypes in human populations encode an HLA-A and/or an HLA-B allotype that has the Bw4 epitope, and consequently, approximately 75% of the human population has the Bw4 epitope, whereas approximately 25% lack the Bw4 epitope.[40] The HLA-A*03 and HLA-A*11 allotypes carry the A3/11 epitope recognized by KIR3DL2; however, the precise specificity of this receptor has not been defined.[62,63] Peptide bound by HLA-A3/11 influences its binding to KIR3DL2,[64] and HLA-A3/11-KIR3DL2 recognition does not seem to educate NK cells.[65] HLA-G, the ligand for KIR2DL4, is expressed only by the extravillous trophoblast (EVT) and is implicated in the interactions between EVT and uterine NK cells, which are critical for placentation and successful reproduction.[66,67] In addition to its activation function, the KIR2DL4 carries a single ITIM in its cytoplasmic tail and exhibits inhibitory function.[68,69]

Although the specificity of the inhibitory KIR have been extensively characterized, very little is known about the ligands for the activating KIRs. Activating KIRs display a high degree of sequence homology with the corresponding inhibitory KIR in their extracellular Ig domains and therefore are predicted to bind to the same HLA class I ligands as their structurally related inhibitory KIRs. For instance, 3DS1 that shares the highest sequence homologies with 3DL1 in their extracellular portion is believed to bind to HLA-Bw4.[70] Whereas KIR2DL1 and 2DS1 differ by only 7 amino acids in their extracellular portion, KIR2DL1 binds to HLA-C2 much more strongly than KIR2DS1.[45,71–74] Similarly, KIR2DL2 and 2DL3 bind to HLA-C1, but KIR2DS2, whose extracellular domain differs from KIR2DL2 and 2DL3 by only 3 and 4 amino acids, respectively, failed to bind any HLA class I molecule examined.[45] The oldest and most prevalent activating receptor KIR2DS4 recognizes some C1- or C2-bearing HLA-C allotypes, as well as the HLA-A3/11 epitope.[50,75] Three other activating KIRs (2DS2, 2DS3, and 2DS5) once recognized HLA-C, but during the course of human evolution they have acquired mutations that block this function.[50,75] Taken as a whole, an intact HLA class I trimer, composed of heavy chain, β2-microglobulin, and peptide, is required for KIR recognition.

CLONAL EXPRESSION OF KILLER CELL IMMUNOGLOBULIN-LIKE RECEPTORS AND ACQUISITION OF NATURAL KILLER CELL TOLERANCE AND RESPONSIVENESS

Like T and B lymphocytes, NK cells are developed from CD34[+] hematopoietic stem cells in the bone marrow and undergo terminal maturation in secondary lymphoid tissues.[76] KIRs are clonally expressed on mature NK cells, so that each NK cell clone expresses only a portion of the genes within the gene profile in an apparently random combination[65,77,78] (Fig. 4). Stochastic expression of different combinations of receptors by NK cells results in this repertoire of NK clones with a variety of ligand specificities, which presumably are critical for a rapid and sensitive detection of reduced HLA class I expression on target cells. Once a given KIR is expressed on an NK cell clone or T cell, it is stably maintained in the progeny of the clone. This pattern of expression seems to be epigenetically regulated by DNA methylation and histone modifications,[79] as well as noncoding RNAs located in the KIR locus.[80] Furthermore, the presence of the cognate HLA class I ligand is shown to increase the frequency of NK cells expressing the specific inhibitory KIR.[44] Finally, a recent study indicates an unexpected and strong epistatic influence on the expression of one KIR (KIR2DL1) by other KIRs (2DL2 and 2DS2).[78]

Most NK cells in peripheral blood express at least one inhibitory receptor for self-MHC class I and are functionally competent to recognize and eliminate target cells that have downregulated their respective MHC class I ligands.[77,81] In addition, a subpopulation of developmentally immature NK cells exists that lacks inhibitory receptors for self-MHC class I and is generally hyporesponsive to target cells that are deficient in MHC class I expression.[82,83] Developmental interactions of the KIRs with HLA class I trigger the acquisition of functional competence in a process called 'licensing',[83,84] 'arming'[85] or 'education'.[82] Therefore, individuals carry a minimum of one inhibitory KIR-HLA gene pair, crucial for the development of functional NK cells.[86] Consistent with this, the NK cells from MHC-deficient mice and humans are shown to be defective in target killing.[87,88] Expression of progressively higher numbers of inhibitory KIRs for self-HLA-B and HLA-Cw molecules has been correlated with an increased effector capacity.[89] In summary, interactions of KIR to HLA class I ligands set the threshold of NK cell capacity as well as control the NK cell response.

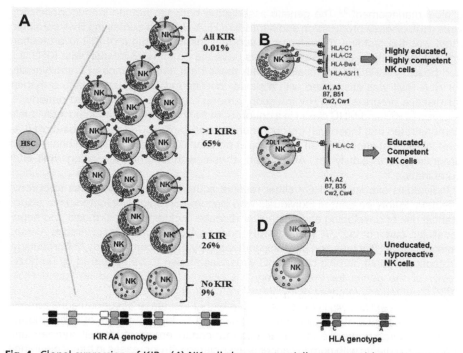

Fig. 4. Clonal expression of KIRs. (*A*) NK cell clones potentially generated from the hematopoietic stem cell (HSC) of an individual carrying simple AA KIR genotype (haplotype A homozygote). Each NK cell clone expresses only a portion of the genes within the KIR genotype that individual carries. Most of the NK cells in AA homozygotes express more than one receptor, whereas ~26% express a single KIR. Approximately 9% of NK cells lack all KIRs, whereas cells expressing all KIRs comprise less than 0.01%. The functional capacity of NK cells is determined based on the availability of cognate HLA class I ligands. For example, if the individual expresses all 4 known HLA class I ligands (*B*), that individual potentially generate highly competent NK cells because of 4 inhibitory KIR and HLA class I interaction–mediated licensing. On the other hand, if the individual carries a single HLA class I ligand (*C*), that individual generates least competent NK cells because of a single inhibitory KIR and HLA class I ligand–mediated licensing. If the NK clones do not express an inhibitory KIR, or express inhibitory KIRs that are not specific to self-HLA class ligands, those NK clones will remain uneducated and hyporesponsive (*D*).

DIVERSITY OF KILLER CELL IMMUNOGLOBULIN-LIKE RECEPTOR–HUMAN LEUKOCYTE ANTIGEN COMPOUND GENOTYPES AND ITS RELEVANCE IN DISEASE

Given that KIR genes at chromosome 19 and HLA genes at chromosome 6 are polymorphic and display significant variations, the independent segregation of these unlinked gene families produce diversity in the number and type of KIR-HLA pairs inherited in individuals,[86] which could influence the health and disease status of a given individual. Consistent with this theory, combinations of certain KIR-HLA genes have been associated with diseases as diverse as autoimmunity, infection, cancer, and reproductive failure.[90–92]

NK cells play a critical role in successful resolution of viral infections in both mice and humans.[93,94] The clearest demonstration of the value of NK cells to humans derives from their deficiency, which represents a small but increasingly appreciated subset of primary immunodeficiencies that present challenges both in diagnosis and clinical management.[95] The genetic association between human immunodeficiency virus (HIV) disease progression and number of HLA-B alleles containing Bw4 serologic motif was the first line of evidence to suggest the involvement of KIR in protection against the virus, because Bw4 allotypes have the potential to interact with KIR3DL1 and possibly KIR3DS1.[70] Consistent with these data, the presence of homozygosity for HLA-Bw4 was associated with a slower decline in CD4+ T-cell count, a marker for disease progression in HIV infection, among a group of HIV-infected patients.[96] Analysis of KIR and MHC class I in a cohort of more than 1000 HIV-infected individuals demonstrated that those with the compound genotype KIR3DS1 and a subset of HLA-Bw4 alleles that encode for an isoleucine at position 80 of the MHC class I heavy chain progress more slowly to AIDS than those without this activating KIR–HLA combination.[97]

Individuals exposed to HCV either resolve acute infection or progress to chronic infection. Eighty percent of individuals who become chronically infected have a substantial risk of developing end-stage liver disease, including liver cirrhosis and hepatocellular carcinoma.[98] A role for KIR and HLA genotypes in clearance versus persistence of HCV infection has been indicated by a multicenter study.[99] Particularly, protection against chronic hepatitis C virus was shown to be conferred by homozygosity of the genes for the inhibitory NK receptor KIR2DL3 and its ligand HLA-C^{Asn80}, particularly in cases of low inoculum of virus.[99]

Elimination of NK cells in mice results in a higher incidence of spontaneous tumors, impaired clearance of inoculated tumor cells, and an increased rate of tumor metastasis.[100] A large body of evidence argues that enhancement of NK cell numbers and function in patients with human cancer is associated with increases in tumor clearance and duration of clinical remission.[101] KIRs seem to influence malignancies, specifically those associated with viral infections. Women developing cervical carcinoma are more likely to express KIR and HLA genotypes associated with activation,[102] whereas reduced susceptibility to hepatocellular carcinoma is associated with activating KIR and HLA allotypes.[103]

Although the cell surface expression and ligands for activating KIRs have not been clearly defined, a series of genetic epidemiologic data have revealed the association of distinct activating KIR in autoimmune diseases. In these models, the activation signals were proposed to prevail over HLA-dependent inhibition that presumably exacerbates NK cell response.[9] KIR2DS2 or 2DS1 were found to be strongly associated with most of the autoimmune conditions. A recent study with Japanese, a highly homogeneous population appropriate for studying genetic associations, found a strong association between the telomeric KIR3DS1-2DL5A-2DS1-2DS5 gene content motif and patients with Vogt-Koyanagi-Harada disease.[104]

HEMATOPOIETIC STEM CELL TRANSPLANTATION

Allogeneic (genetically different) HCT is an effective therapy for an increasing number of life-threatening hematological, oncological, hereditary, and immunologic diseases.[105] Patients undergoing matched unrelated donor HCT, compared with those receiving sibling HCT, display a higher incidence of graft-versus-host disease (GVHD), suggesting the role of non–T cell-mediated mechanisms involved in GVHD and graft-versus-tumor effect. Following allogeneic HST, the progeny of the donor stem cells repopulate the entire hematopoietic system of the recipient. NK cells are the first lymphocyte population to appear in peripheral blood shortly after HST. KIR repertoires of NK cells reconstituted from the donor hematopoietic precursors are consistently of donor type. The donor-derived NK cells can be alloreactive if their inhibitory KIRs do not see a relevant HLA class I ligand that was present in the donor. Such alloreactive NK cells greatly contribute many potential benefits, including (1) decreased rates of GVHD, (2) decreased rates of graft rejection mediated by NK lysis of host T cells, (3) decreased relapse, (4) improved engraftment mediated by NK-cell release of hematopoietic cytokines, and (5) enhanced immune reconstitution and decreased infectious complications mediated by NK-cell antiviral activity. Such beneficial NK-cell alloreactivity, which can be predicted from the differences in KIR-binding HLA class I ligands between donor and recipient based on their HLA class I type, was first described for HLA haploidentical transplantation by the use of an extensively T-cell–depleted graft in acute myeloid leukemia (AML) patients and later investigated in other transplantation settings.[106]

In addition to the recipient lacking HLA class I ligands for the donor-derived NK cells, expression of activating KIRs on donor NK cells is also shown to influence HST outcome, particularly in HLA-matched HST setting. Compared with donors with AA genotypes (express one or no activating KIR), the Bx genotype (express 1–6 activating KIRs) donors were shown to contribute significantly superior relapse protection and improved disease-free survival for AML patients.[107–110] Gene content motif analyses further reveal that the centromeric and telomeric B haplotype-specific motifs both contribute to relapse protection and improved survival. In summary, knowing the KIR genotype of the donor, and HLA types of both the donor and recipient, it is possible to predict the degree of KIR-HLA interactions that may determine an enhanced ability to limit GVHD and improve engraftment for certain types of leukemia.

SUMMARY

NK cells are more than simple killers and have been implicated in control and clearance of malignant and virally infected cells, regulation of adaptive immune responses, rejection of bone marrow transplants, autoimmunity, and the maintenance of pregnancy. The independent segregation of polymorphic KIR and HLA genes results in variable KIR-HLA combinations in individuals, which may determine an individual's immunity and susceptibility to diseases as diverse as autoimmunity, viral infections, and cancer.

REFERENCES

1. Trinchieri G. Biology of natural killer cells. Adv Immunol 1989;47:187–376.
2. Lee SH, Miyagi T, Biron CA. Keeping NK cells in highly regulated antiviral warfare. Trends Immunol 2007;28:252–9.
3. Smyth MJ, Hayakawa Y, Takeda K, et al. New aspects of natural-killer-cell surveillance and therapy of cancer. Nat Rev Cancer 2002;2:850–61.
4. Sun JC, Beilke JN, Lanier LL. Adaptive immune features of natural killer cells. Nature 2009;457:557–61.
5. Gregoire C, Cognet C, Chasson L, et al. Intrasplenic trafficking of natural killer cells is redirected by chemokines upon inflammation. Eur J Immunol 2008;38:2076–84.
6. Colucci F, Caligiuri MA, Di Santo JP. What does it take to make a natural killer? Nat Rev Immunol 2003;3:413–25.
7. Karre K, Ljunggren HG, Piontek G, et al. Selective rejection of H-2-deficient lymphoma variants suggests alternative immune defence strategy. Nature 1986;319:675–8.

8. Ljunggren HG, Karre K. In search of the 'missing self': MHC molecules and NK cell recognition. Immunol Today 1990;11:237–44.
9. Lanier LL. NK cell recognition. Annu Rev Immunol 2005;23:225–74.
10. Bryceson YT, Long EO. Line of attack: NK cell specificity and integration of signals. Curr Opin Immunol 2008;20:344–52.
11. Lanier LL. Natural killer cell receptor signaling. Curr Opin Immunol 2003;15: 308–14.
12. McQueen KL, Parham P. Variable receptors controlling activation and inhibition of NK cells. Curr Opin Immunol 2002;14:615–21.
13. Moretta L, Biassoni R, Bottino C, et al. Human NK-cell receptors. Immunol Today 2000;21:420–2.
14. Vivier E, Raulet DH, Moretta A, et al. Innate or adaptive immunity? The example of natural killer cells. Science 2011;331:44–9.
15. Lanier LL. NK cell receptors. Annu Rev Immunol 1998;16:359–93.
16. Long EO, Barber DF, Burshtyn DN, et al. Inhibition of natural killer cell activation signals by killer cell immunoglobulin-like receptors (CD158). Immunol Rev 2001; 181:223–33.
17. Moretta A, Bottino C, Vitale M, et al. Activating receptors and coreceptors involved in human natural killer cell-mediated cytolysis. Annu Rev Immunol 2001;19:197–223.
18. Vilches C, Parham P. KIR: diverse, rapidly evolving receptors of innate and adaptive immunity. Annu Rev Immunol 2002;20:217–51.
19. Wilson MJ, Torkar M, Haude A, et al. Plasticity in the organization and sequences of human KIR/ILT gene families. Proc Natl Acad Sci U S A 2000;97: 4778–83.
20. Trowsdale J. Genetic and functional relationships between MHC and NK receptor genes. Immunity 2001;15:363–74.
21. Marsh SG, Parham P, Dupont B, et al. Killer-cell immunoglobulin-like receptor (KIR) nomenclature report, 2002. Tissue Antigens 2003;62:79–86.
22. Uhrberg M, Valiante NM, Shum BP, et al. Human diversity in killer cell inhibitory receptor genes. Immunity 1997;7:753–63.
23. Hsu KC, Chida S, Geraghty DE, et al. The killer cell immunoglobulin-like receptor (KIR) genomic region: gene-order, haplotypes and allelic polymorphism. Immunol Rev 2002;190:40–52.
24. Hsu KC, Liu XR, Selvakumar A, et al. Killer Ig-like receptor haplotype analysis by gene content: evidence for genomic diversity with a minimum of six basic framework haplotypes, each with multiple subsets. J Immunol 2002;169:5118–29.
25. Shilling HG, Guethlein LA, Cheng NW, et al. Allelic polymorphism synergizes with variable gene content to individualize human KIR genotype. J Immunol 2002;168:2307–15.
26. Middleton D, Meenagh A, Gourraud PA. KIR haplotype content at the allele level in 77 Northern Irish families. Immunogenetics 2007;59:145–58.
27. Yawata M, Yawata N, Abi-Rached L, et al. Variation within the human killer cell immunoglobulin-like receptor (KIR) gene family. Crit Rev Immunol 2002;22: 463–82.
28. Vierra-Green C, Roe D, Hou L, et al. Allele-level haplotype frequencies and pairwise linkage disequilibrium for 14 KIR loci in 506 European-American individuals. PLoS One 2012;7:e47491.
29. Norman PJ, Abi-Rached L, Gendzekhadze K, et al. Meiotic recombination generates rich diversity in NK cell receptor genes, alleles, and haplotypes. Genome Res 2009;19:757–69.

30. Rajalingam R, Du Z, Meenagh A, et al. Distinct diversity of KIR genes in three southern Indian populations: comparison with world populations revealed a link between KIR gene content and pre-historic human migrations. Immunogenetics 2008;60:207–17.

31. Middleton D, Menchaca L, Rood H, et al. New allele frequency database: http://www.allelefrequencies.net. Tissue Antigens 2003;61:403–7.

32. Jiang K, Zhu FM, Lv QF, et al. Distribution of killer cell immunoglobulin-like receptor genes in the Chinese Han population. Tissue Antigens 2005;65:556–63.

33. Yawata M, Yawata N, McQueen KL, et al. Predominance of group A KIR haplotypes in Japanese associated with diverse NK cell repertoires of KIR expression. Immunogenetics 2002;54:543–50.

34. Whang DH, Park H, Yoon JA, et al. Haplotype analysis of killer cell immunoglobulin-like receptor genes in 77 Korean families. Hum Immunol 2005;66:146–54.

35. Gendzekhadze K, Norman PJ, Abi-Rached L, et al. High KIR diversity in Amerindians is maintained using few gene-content haplotypes. Immunogenetics 2006;58:474–80.

36. Ewerton PD, Leite Mde M, Magalhaes M, et al. Amazonian Amerindians exhibit high variability of KIR profiles. Immunogenetics 2007;59:625–30.

37. Toneva M, Lepage V, Lafay G, et al. Genomic diversity of natural killer cell receptor genes in three populations. Tissue Antigens 2001;57:358–62.

38. Rajalingam R, Krausa P, Shilling HG, et al. Distinctive KIR and HLA diversity in a panel of north Indian Hindus. Immunogenetics 2002;53:1009–19.

39. Kulkarni S, Single RM, Martin MP, et al. Comparison of the rapidly evolving KIR locus in Parsis and natives of India. Immunogenetics 2008;60:121–9.

40. Norman PJ, Abi-Rached L, Gendzekhadze K, et al. Unusual selection on the KIR3DL1/S1 natural killer cell receptor in Africans. Nat Genet 2007;39:1092–9.

41. Gardiner CM, Guethlein LA, Shilling HG, et al. Different NK cell surface phenotypes defined by the DX9 antibody are due to KIR3DL1 gene polymorphism. J Immunol 2001;166:2992–3001.

42. Jones DC, Hiby SE, Moffett A, et al. Nature of allelic sequence polymorphism at the KIR3DL3 locus. Immunogenetics 2006;58:614–27.

43. Hou L, Chen M, Steiner NK, et al. Seventeen novel alleles add to the already extensive KIR3DL3 diversity. Tissue Antigens 2007;70:449–54.

44. Yawata M, Yawata N, Draghi M, et al. Roles for HLA and KIR polymorphisms in natural killer cell repertoire selection and modulation of effector function. J Exp Med 2006;203:633–45.

45. Winter CC, Gumperz JE, Parham P, et al. Direct binding and functional transfer of NK cell inhibitory receptors reveal novel patterns of HLA-C allotype recognition. J Immunol 1998;161:571–7.

46. VandenBussche CJ, Dakshanamurthy S, Posch PE, et al. A single polymorphism disrupts the killer Ig-like receptor 2DL2/2DL3 D1 domain. J Immunol 2006;177:5347–57.

47. O'Connor GM, Guinan KJ, Cunningham RT, et al. Functional polymorphism of the KIR3DL1/S1 receptor on human NK cells. J Immunol 2007;178:235–41.

48. Carr WH, Pando MJ, Parham P. KIR3DL1 polymorphisms that affect NK cell inhibition by HLA-Bw4 ligand. J Immunol 2005;175:5222–9.

49. Bari R, Bell T, Leung WH, et al. Significant functional heterogeneity among KIR2DL1 alleles and a pivotal role of arginine 245. Blood 2009;114:5182–90.

50. Hilton HG, Vago L, Older Aguilar AM, et al. Mutation at positively selected positions in the binding site for HLA-C shows that KIR2DL1 is a more refined but less adaptable NK cell receptor than KIR2DL3. J Immunol 2012;189:1418–30.

51. Steiner NK, Dakshanamurthy S, Nguyen N, et al. Allelic variation of killer cell immunoglobulin-like receptor 2DS5 impacts glycosylation altering cell surface expression levels. Hum Immunol 2014;75:124–8.

52. Pando MJ, Gardiner CM, Gleimer M, et al. The protein made from a common allele of KIR3DL1 (3DL1*004) is poorly expressed at cell surfaces due to substitution at positions 86 in Ig domain 0 and 182 in Ig domain 1. J Immunol 2003; 171:6640–9.

53. Klein J, Sato A. The HLA system. Second of two parts. N Engl J Med 2000;343: 782–6.

54. Klein J, Sato A. The HLA system. First of two parts. N Engl J Med 2000;343: 702–9.

55. Colonna M, Spies T, Strominger JL, et al. Alloantigen recognition by two human natural killer cell clones is associated with HLA-C or a closely linked gene. Proc Natl Acad Sci U S A 1992;89:7983–5.

56. Colonna M, Borsellino G, Falco M, et al. HLA-C is the inhibitory ligand that determines dominant resistance to lysis by NK1- and NK2-specific natural killer cells. Proc Natl Acad Sci U S A 1993;90:12000–4.

57. Wagtmann N, Biassoni R, Cantoni C, et al. Molecular clones of the p58 NK cell receptor reveal immunoglobulin-related molecules with diversity in both the extra- and intracellular domains. Immunity 1995;2:439–49.

58. Winter CC, Long EO. A single amino acid in the p58 killer cell inhibitory receptor controls the ability of natural killer cells to discriminate between the two groups of HLA-C allotypes. J Immunol 1997;158:4026–8.

59. Gumperz JE, Litwin V, Phillips JH, et al. The Bw4 public epitope of HLA-B molecules confers reactivity with natural killer cell clones that express NKB1, a putative HLA receptor. J Exp Med 1995;181:1133–44.

60. Cella M, Longo A, Ferrara GB, et al. NK3-specific natural killer cells are selectively inhibited by Bw4-positive HLA alleles with isoleucine 80. J Exp Med 1994;180:1235–42.

61. Thananchai H, Gillespie G, Martin MP, et al. Cutting edge: allele-specific and peptide-dependent interactions between KIR3DL1 and HLA-A and HLA-B. J Immunol 2007;178:33–7.

62. Pende D, Biassoni R, Cantoni C, et al. The natural killer cell receptor specific for HLA-A allotypes: a novel member of the p58/p70 family of inhibitory receptors that is characterized by three immunoglobulin-like domains and is expressed as a 140-kD disulphide-linked dimer. J Exp Med 1996;184:505–18.

63. Dohring C, Scheidegger D, Samaridis J, et al. A human killer inhibitory receptor specific for HLA-A1,2. J Immunol 1996;156:3098–101.

64. Hansasuta P, Dong T, Thananchai H, et al. Recognition of HLA-A3 and HLA-A11 by KIR3DL2 is peptide-specific. Eur J Immunol 2004;34:1673–9.

65. Yawata M, Yawata N, Draghi M, et al. MHC class I-specific inhibitory receptors and their ligands structure diverse human NK-cell repertoires toward a balance of missing self-response. Blood 2008;112:2369–80.

66. Moffett A, Colucci F. Co-evolution of NK receptors and HLA ligands in humans is driven by reproduction. Immunol Rev 2015;267:283–97.

67. Rajagopalan S, Bryceson YT, Kuppusamy SP, et al. Activation of NK cells by an endocytosed receptor for soluble HLA-G. PLoS Biol 2006;4:e9.

68. Faure M, Long EO. KIR2DL4 (CD158d), an NK cell-activating receptor with inhibitory potential. J Immunol 2002;168:6208–14.
69. Yusa S, Catina TL, Campbell KS. SHP-1- and phosphotyrosine-independent inhibitory signaling by a killer cell Ig-like receptor cytoplasmic domain in human NK cells. J Immunol 2002;168:5047–57.
70. Carrington M, O'Brien SJ. The influence of HLA genotype on AIDS. Annu Rev Med 2003;54:535–51.
71. Sivori S, Carlomagno S, Falco M, et al. Natural killer cells expressing the KIR2DS1-activating receptor efficiently kill T-cell blasts and dendritic cells: implications in haploidentical HSCT. Blood 2011;117:4284–92.
72. Chewning JH, Gudme CN, Hsu KC, et al. KIR2DS1-positive NK cells mediate alloresponse against the C2 HLA-KIR ligand group in vitro. J Immunol 2007; 179:854–68.
73. Moesta AK, Abi-Rached L, Norman PJ, et al. Chimpanzees use more varied receptors and ligands than humans for inhibitory killer cell Ig-like receptor recognition of the MHC-C1 and MHC-C2 epitopes. J Immunol 2009;182:3628–37.
74. Stewart CA, Laugier-Anfossi F, Vely F, et al. Recognition of peptide-MHC class I complexes by activating killer immunoglobulin-like receptors. Proc Natl Acad Sci U S A 2005;102:13224–9.
75. Saulquin X, Gastinel LN, Vivier E. Crystal structure of the human natural killer cell activating receptor KIR2DS2 (CD158j). J Exp Med 2003;197:933–8.
76. Montaldo E, Del Zotto G, Della Chiesa M, et al. Human NK cell receptors/markers: a tool to analyze NK cell development, subsets and function. Cytometry A 2013;83:702–13.
77. Valiante NM, Uhrberg M, Shilling HG, et al. Functionally and structurally distinct NK cell receptor repertoires in the peripheral blood of two human donors. Immunity 1997;7:739–51.
78. Schonberg K, Sribar M, Enczmann J, et al. Analyses of HLA-C-specific KIR repertoires in donors with group A and B haplotypes suggest a ligand-instructed model of NK cell receptor acquisition. Blood 2011;117:98–107.
79. Santourlidis S, Graffmann N, Christ J, et al. Lineage-specific transition of histone signatures in the killer cell Ig-like receptor locus from hematopoietic progenitor to NK cells. J Immunol 2008;180:418–25.
80. Cichocki F, Lenvik T, Sharma N, et al. Cutting edge: KIR antisense transcripts are processed into a 28-base PIWI-like RNA in human NK cells. J Immunol 2010;185:2009–12.
81. Raulet DH, Vance RE, McMahon CW. Regulation of the natural killer cell receptor repertoire. Annu Rev Immunol 2001;19:291–330.
82. Anfossi N, Andre P, Guia S, et al. Human NK cell education by inhibitory receptors for MHC class I. Immunity 2006;25(2):331–42.
83. Kim S, Poursine-Laurent J, Truscott SM, et al. Licensing of natural killer cells by host major histocompatibility complex class I molecules. Nature 2005;436: 709–13.
84. Yokoyama WM, Kim S. How do natural killer cells find self to achieve tolerance? Immunity 2006;24:249–57.
85. Raulet DH, Vance RE. Self-tolerance of natural killer cells. Nat Rev Immunol 2006;6:520–31.
86. Du Z, Gjertson DW, Reed EF, et al. Receptor-ligand analyses define minimal killer cell Ig-like receptor (KIR) in humans. Immunogenetics 2007;59:1–15.
87. Bix M, Liao NS, Zijlstra M, et al. Rejection of class I MHC-deficient haemopoietic cells by irradiated MHC-matched mice. Nature 1991;349:329–31.

88. Furukawa H, Yabe T, Watanabe K, et al. Tolerance of NK and LAK activity for HLA class I-deficient targets in a TAP1-deficient patient (bare lymphocyte syndrome type I). Hum Immunol 1999;60:32–40.
89. Yu J, Heller G, Chewning J, et al. Hierarchy of the human natural killer cell response is determined by class and quantity of inhibitory receptors for self-HLA-B and HLA-C ligands. J Immunol 2007;179:5977–89.
90. Khakoo SI, Carrington M. KIR and disease: a model system or system of models? Immunol Rev 2006;214:186–201.
91. Kulkarni S, Martin MP, Carrington M. The Yin and Yang of HLA and KIR in human disease. Semin Immunol 2008;20:343–52.
92. Rajalingam R. Human diversity of killer cell immunoglobulin-like receptors and disease. Korean J Hematol 2011;46:216–28.
93. Biron CA, Nguyen KB, Pien GC, et al. Natural killer cells in antiviral defense: function and regulation by innate cytokines. Annu Rev Immunol 1999;17: 189–220.
94. Orange JS, Ballas ZK. Natural killer cells in human health and disease. Clin Immunol 2006;118:1–10.
95. Orange JS. Natural killer cell deficiency. J Allergy Clin Immunol 2013;132: 515–25 [quiz: 26].
96. Flores-Villanueva PO, Yunis EJ, Delgado JC, et al. Control of HIV-1 viremia and protection from AIDS are associated with HLA-Bw4 homozygosity. Proc Natl Acad Sci U S A 2001;98:5140–5.
97. Martin MP, Gao X, Lee JH, et al. Epistatic interaction between KIR3DS1 and HLA-B delays the progression to AIDS. Nat Genet 2002;31:429–34.
98. Alter HJ, Seeff LB. Recovery, persistence, and sequelae in hepatitis C virus infection: a perspective on long-term outcome. Semin Liver Dis 2000;20:17–35.
99. Khakoo SI, Thio CL, Martin MP, et al. HLA and NK cell inhibitory receptor genes in resolving hepatitis C virus infection. Science 2004;305:872–4.
100. Waldhauer I, Steinle A. NK cells and cancer immunosurveillance. Oncogene 2008;27:5932–43.
101. Zamai L, Ponti C, Mirandola P, et al. NK cells and cancer. J Immunol 2007;178: 4011–6.
102. Carrington M, Wang S, Martin MP, et al. Hierarchy of resistance to cervical neoplasia mediated by combinations of killer immunoglobulin-like receptor and human leukocyte antigen loci. J Exp Med 2005;201:1069–75.
103. Lopez-Vazquez A, Rodrigo L, Martinez-Borra J, et al. Protective effect of the HLA-Bw4I80 epitope and the killer cell immunoglobulin-like receptor 3DS1 gene against the development of hepatocellular carcinoma in patients with hepatitis C virus infection. J Infect Dis 2005;192:162–5.
104. Levinson RD, Okada AA, Ashouri E, et al. Killer cell immunoglobulin-like receptor gene-cluster 3DS1-2DL5-2DS1-2DS5 predisposes susceptibility to Vogt-Koyanagi-Harada syndrome in Japanese individuals. Hum Immunol 2010;71: 192–4.
105. Appelbaum FR. The current status of hematopoietic cell transplantation. Annu Rev Med 2003;54:491–512.
106. Ruggeri L, Capanni M, Urbani E, et al. Effectiveness of donor natural killer cell alloreactivity in mismatched hematopoietic transplants. Science 2002;295: 2097–100.
107. Cooley S, Trachtenberg E, Bergemann TL, et al. Donors with group B KIR haplotypes improve relapse-free survival after unrelated hematopoietic cell transplantation for acute myelogenous leukemia. Blood 2009;113:726–32.

108. Hsu KC, Gooley T, Malkki M, et al. KIR ligands and prediction of relapse after unrelated donor hematopoietic cell transplantation for hematologic malignancy. Biol Blood Marrow Transplant 2006;12:828–36.

109. Stringaris K, Adams S, Uribe M, et al. Donor KIR genes 2DL5A, 2DS1 and 3DS1 are associated with a reduced rate of leukaemia relapse after HLA-identical sibling stem cell transplantation for acute myeloid Leukaemia but not other haematological malignancies. Biol Blood Marrow Transplant 2010;16(9):1257–64.

110. Cooley S, Weisdorf DJ, Guethlein LA, et al. Donor selection for natural killer cell receptor genes leads to superior survival after unrelated transplantation for acute myelogenous leukemia. Blood 2010;116:2411–9.

The Role of Human Leukocyte Antigen in Celiac Disease Diagnostics

Eszter Lázár-Molnár, PhD[a],*, Melissa Snyder, PhD[b]

KEYWORDS

● Celiac disease ● HLA-DQ2 ● HLA-DQ8 ● Disease association

KEY POINTS

● Celiac disease is an immune-mediated gastrointestinal disease caused by exposure to cereal gluten in genetically susceptible individuals.

● Genetic risk for celiac disease includes the presence of HLA-DQ2 or HLA-DQ8, which are major players in pathogenesis by their ability to present pathogenic gluten peptides and trigger an immune response.

● Diagnostic tools include intestinal biopsy and detection of antibodies to deamidated gliadin peptides and tissue transglutaminase. Serologies may be affected by immunoglobulin A deficiency or gluten-free diet.

● Genetic testing for HLA-DQ2 and DQ8 is useful in ruling out celiac disease diagnosis. Although a positive test is generally not diagnostic for celiac disease, recent guidelines place more emphasis on HLA testing in the context of specific pediatric patient populations.

INTRODUCTION

Celiac disease (CD) is an immune-mediated chronic gastrointestinal (GI) disease affecting the small intestine. CD development is influenced by both environmental and genetic factors. The disease was first described by the Greek physician Aretaeus in ancient Rome[1] but it was not until the 1950s, when its causal role was discovered. The environmental factor that leads to CD has been conclusively identified when Willem Karel Dicke, a Dutch pediatrician, demonstrated the causal role of dietary gluten and proposed to treat patients by life-long gluten-free diet (GFD).[2] Gluten is a cereal grain protein found in wheat; related proteins, also associated with CD, are found in barley and rye. In genetically susceptible individuals, ingestion of these cereal grains leads to an inflammatory response in the small intestine. CD is a polygenic

Disclosure Statement: The authors have nothing to disclose.
[a] ARUP Laboratories, Department of Pathology, University of Utah School of Medicine, 500 Chipeta Way, MS 115, Salt Lake City, UT 84108, USA; [b] Department of Laboratory Medicine and Pathology, Mayo Clinic, 200 First Street Southwest, Rochester, MN 55905, USA
* Corresponding author. ARUP Laboratories, 500 Chipeta Way, MS115, Salt Lake City, UT 84108.
E-mail address: eszter.lazar-molnar@aruplab.com

Clin Lab Med 38 (2018) 655–668
https://doi.org/10.1016/j.cll.2018.07.007
0272-2712/18/© 2018 Elsevier Inc. All rights reserved.

labmed.theclinics.com

disorder, meaning that many genes contribute to an individual's overall genetic susceptibility to developing the disease. However, the strongest genetic association that seems to be critical for the pathogenesis of the disease is the presence of human leukocyte antigens HLA-DQ2 or HLA-DQ8. Studies have demonstrated that virtually all individuals with CD are positive for either one or both of these of HLA molecules. This critical association is borne out in the mechanism of CD. When gluten is digested, certain peptides are produced, which display high affinity for the HLA-DQ2 or HLA-DQ8 molecules. The HLA/peptide complex will then be recognized by T cells possessing specific T-cell receptor (TCR). Engagement of the TCR leads to activation and proliferation of the T cells, subsequently followed by antibody production through B cell–derived plasma cells, and ultimately the inflammatory response within the GI tract that is associated with this disorder.

Although awareness of CD seems to be on the rise, establishing a diagnosis can still be challenging. This may be due, in part, to the wide variety of symptoms with which patients may present. Although some symptoms, such as abdominal pain, steatorrhea, and weight loss, are clearly linked to a GI pathology, many symptoms are not so obvious. In fact, many patients are evaluated for CD based on non-GI symptoms, including fatigue, arthralgia, infertility, and neurologic manifestations. As a result, initial testing for CD is often performed outside of the care of a gastroenterologist.

The complexity of testing for CD is another diagnostic challenge. Historically, CD diagnoses were based almost exclusively on the small-intestinal biopsy. The presence of certain features on the biopsy, in conjunction with clinical evaluation, could be sufficient to support the diagnosis of CD. However, there are certain drawbacks to the biopsy approach, namely that it is an invasive procedure with certain risks and may not be tolerated or desired by some patients. Fortunately, the antibody production that occurs as part of the pathogenesis provides an important tool for the diagnosis of CD, after the demonstration in the 1970s that CD is specifically associated with autoantibodies to a tissue antigen.[3] More recently, major advance in serologic testing have begun to lessen our reliance on biopsy. Patients with CD can produce antibodies to a variety of target antigens. One antigen in particular, gliadin, is directly related to the environmental cause of CD, the dietary gluten. As part of the inflammatory response, patients with CD may develop antibodies to gliadin, either modified or unmodified. As the immune response evolves, patients can develop antibodies to autoantigens, including tissue transglutaminase (TTG). Although all of these markers can be used diagnostically, there are also some characteristics that limit their applicability in certain patients.

In addition to serology, genetic testing specifically for HLA-DQ2 and HLA-DQ8 can play a role in diagnosis. Although not necessarily required, there are certain situations where the negative predictive value of this test can be used to "rule out" the diagnosis. The remainder of this article examines in more detail how biopsy, serology, and genetic testing can be used to most accurately and efficiently evaluate patients with suspected CD.

GENETICS OF CELIAC DISEASE

The mechanism of CD development is an interplay between both environmental and genetic factors. The most important environmental factor in the development of CD is gluten consumption, which is reflected in the worldwide distribution of CD, being prevalent in countries where wheat is a major part of the diet. Genetic susceptibility is, however, a key factor, because only individuals with predisposing genetic background will develop the disease. Environmental factors in the context of genetic susceptibility trigger the immune system, which is the root cause of CD pathogenesis.

The most important genetic factor in CD development is the presence of specific HLA Class II molecules HLA-DQ2 or HLA-DQ8, which has been shown to account to up to 40% of genetic risk.[4] In addition to CD, the presence of the DR3-DQ2 and DR4-DQ8 haplotypes is also associated with other autoimmune diseases such as type I diabetes (T1D).

Associations of the HLA alleles encoding for HLA-DQ2 and DQ8 heterodimers with CD represent one of the strongest HLA disease associations discovered.[5] Ninety to ninety-five percent of patients with CD express a particular HLA-DQ2 heterodimer molecule encoded by HLA-DQA1*05 allele in combination with HLA-DQB1*02 allele, also referred to as HLA-DQ2.5 (**Fig. 1**). This heterodimer can be encoded in *cis* arrangement, when both alleles are located on the same chromosome, present in individuals who have the HLA-DQA1*05:01/HLA-DQB1*02:01 haplotype. This haplotype is also commonly associated with HLA-DR3 and is referred to as DR3-DQ2 haplotype. The HLA-DQ2.5 heterodimer can also be encoded by alleles in *trans* arrangement in those who express HLA-DQA1*05:05 with HLA-DQB1*03:01 (DQ7) on one chromosome, also associated with DR5 (DR5-DQ7 haplotype), and DQB1*02:02 with DQA1*02:01 on the other chromosome, associated with DR7 (DR7-DQ2 haplotype). The DQ alpha chains encoded by DQA1*05:01 and DQA1*05:05 differ by only one residue in the leader peptide; similarly, the DQ beta chains encoded by DQB1*02:01 and DQB1*02:02 differ by only one residue in the membrane proximal domain; it is unlikely that those differences would have any functional consequence because they do not affect the chemistry of the peptide-binding domain.[6] Because of the codominant expression of HLA, the heterodimer associated with CD will be able to form in both *cis* (both alpha and beta chains being part of the same haplotype) and *trans* (alpha and beta chains part of different haplotypes) arrangement of the alleles.

In addition to HLA-DQ2, 5% to 10% of the patients with CD carry HLA-DQ8 encoded by HLA-DQB1*03:02 allele, most commonly in combination with HLA-DQA1*03:01, and also associated with DR4 (DR4-DQ8 haplotype). Certain individuals may be heterozygous for DR4-DQ8 and DR3-DQ2.5 haplotypes, which confers additional risk compared with DR4-DQ8 in association with a nonrisk haplotype. Of interest, the presence of heterozygous HLA-DQ2.5 and DQ8 also predisposes to T1D with an almost 5-fold higher risk than those who are homozygous to either variant,

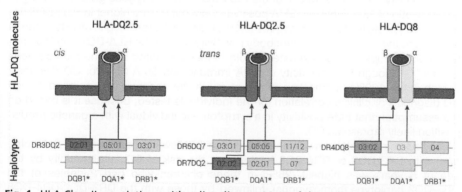

Fig. 1. HLA Class II associations with celiac disease. Most of the patients with celiac disease (90%) express the HLA-DQ2.5 heterodimer, which consists of the combination HLA DQA1*05 and DQB1*02 alleles in either *cis* configuration on the same DR3-DQ2 haplotype or in *trans* configuration, located on different chromosomes (DR5-DQ7 and DR7-DQ2 haplotypes). The remaining patients (5%–10%) express HLA-DQ8 encoded by the HLA DQB1*03:02 allele, typically in combination with DQA1*03 allele within the DR4-DQ8 haplotype.

due to the formation of HLA-DQ8 transdimers between HLA-DQA1*05:01 and HLA-DQB1*03:02.[7]

Patients negative for both HLA-DQ2.5 and DQ8 mostly carry HLA-DQB1*02:02 with HLA-DQA1*02:01 haplotype (HLA-DQ2.2), which has an inconsequential risk for the development of CD.[8] HLA-DQ2.2 confers a much lesser risk than HLA-DQ2.5 because of the replacement of a tyrosine by a phenylalanine in DQ alpha chain at position 22, which is important for peptide binding.[9]

HLA-DQ2 and HLA-DQ8 are necessary but not sufficient for the development of CD. This is also reflected by the much higher representation of these alleles in the general population, in contrast to relatively low CD frequency. Twenty to thirty percent of Caucasians, 20% of African Americans, and 15% to 20% of Hispanics express HLA-DQ2, whereas the frequency of CD is much lower in the general population, showing on average of about 1% prevalence worldwide[10] and in the United States.[11] This incomplete penetrance, even when both genetic predisposition through HLA and environmental factors such as gluten consumption are present, suggests that there could be additional triggers for disease development, which remain to be identified. Viral/bacterial infections, cessation of smoking, changes of lifestyle, changes in intestinal microbiome, and many other factors have been suspected but not necessarily proved to show association with CD development.[12]

HLA Copy Number and Risk

A strong gene dose effect has been observed for HLA-DQ2.5, whereas individuals homozygous for HLA-DQ2.5 are at higher risk for developing CD compared with heterozygous individuals.[13–15] In addition, HLA-DQ2.5 homozygous patients have been shown to have a more severe disease course; this can be explained by a more superior peptide presentation through the antigen-presenting cells expressing the homozygous HLA-DQ2.5, in contrast to heterozygous HLA-DQ2.5, measured by increased T-cell proliferation and cytokine secretion.[15]

In a large study cohort of more than 10,000 US subjects at risk for CD, homozygosity to HLA-DQ2 (either HLA-DQ2.5 homozygous or HLA-DQ2.5/DQ2.2) dramatically increased risk for CD autoimmunity, evaluated as positivity for endomysial antibodies (EMA).[16] Twenty-eight percent of subjects with DQ2 homozygous haplotype showed EMA positivity, in contrast to 9% of the HLA-DQ2.5 heterozygous group, resulting in an odds ratio of 3.94. Similarly, EMA positivity was found to be higher in HLA-DQ8 homozygous (8.4%) versus heterozygous (2.1%) individuals, resulting in an odds ratio of 4.27. Thus, the odds of CD autoantibody positivity among the HLA-DQ2 and DQ8 homozygous groups are approximately 4-fold higher compared with the heterozygous groups.[16] Although the specificity of EMA immunoglobulin A (IgA) for CD diagnosis is high (94%–100%), a limitation of the study is the absence of biopsy-confirmed CD diagnosis or clinical correlation for the individuals tested, because it is based on the assumption that EMA positivity in a symptomatic individual with a genetic predisposition likely represents CD.

In a recent prospective multicenter study for CD development involving 6403 children with DR3-DQ2 or DR4-DQ8 haplotypes, the risk of CD autoimmunity by the age of 5 years was highest (26%) in those children who had 2 copies of the DR3-DQ2 haplotype (homozygous), followed by those with the DR3-DQ2/DR4-DQ8 haplotype (11%).[17] The risk was also higher for those homozygous for DR4-DQ8 haplotype (9%) compared with the heterozygous DR4-DDQ2 haplotype (2%). This resulted in a hazard ratio of 5.7 for CD autoimmunity for the DR3-DQ2 homozygous group, in contrast to 2.09 for the lowest risk DR4-DQ8 genotype group. In addition to CD autoimmunity, which was defined as the presence of serum antibodies against

TTG on 2 consecutive tests at least 3 months apart, CD development was also evaluated, defined by positive intestinal biopsy, or in the absence of biopsy, by persistently high levels of TTG antibodies (TTG antibodies 100 units or higher on consecutive tests). The risk of CD development by the age of 5 years was 11% in the DR3-DQ2 homozygous group, in contrast to 3% in children with a single DR3-DQ2 haplotype.[17]

Non-HLA Genetic Associations

HLA-DQ2 and DQ8 are estimated to contribute up to 40% to the genetic susceptibility to CD.[18] These HLA genes are located in a large haplotype with strong linkage disequilibrium characteristic to HLA, suggesting that other genes associated with the locus may also provide risk.[19] The likely role of non-HLA genes in CD development in addition to HLA-DQ2 and DQ8 are shown by higher concordance rate (70%) between monozygotic twins compared with dizygotic twins (10%).[20]

Recent genome-wide association studies (GWAS) provided additional evidence for association of CD with non-HLA loci. Two GWAS[18,21] and follow-up studies on more than 12,000 patients with CD identified together with the HLA locus a total of 43 loci known to contribute to CD susceptibility.[22] CD-predisposing genetic risk variants included interleukin 2 (IL-2), IL-21, CD28, CTLA4, ICOS, and other genes involved in regulation of T-cell– and B-cell–mediated immune responses, as well as innate responses, intestinal permeability, and others.[23] Of interest, many of the non-HLA risk genes were also implicated in the pathogenesis of other autoimmune conditions such as T1D and rheumatoid arthritis.

The non-HLA loci comprise mainly common single-nucleotide polymorphisms (SNPs), which account for ~15% of the additional genetic risk. The vast majority of CD-associated SNPs does not map on exons but rather intersect with promoter and enhancer sequences in the genome, implying that deregulating expression of genes encoding proteins or regulatory RNAs such as micro RNAs and long noncoding RNAs may govern disease development. Although the causative genes within these loci remain to be identified, most of the candidate genes are implicated in regulation of immune responses,[22] and many of them are also associated with other autoimmune diseases such as rheumatoid arthritis and T1D.

The Role of HLA in Immune Mechanism to Celiac Disease

The HLA-DQ2.5 molecules predispose to CD by preferential presentation of gluten antigens to CD4+ T cells. Although HLA-DQ2.5 heterodimer predisposes to CD, HLA-DQ2.2 does not, which is explained by the ability of DQ2.5 to present a larger repertoire of gluten peptides, whereas the DQ2.2 can only present a subset of them.[15] In addition, HLA-DQ2.5 was found to have greater stability of bound peptides as opposed to HLA-DQ2.2, enabling sustained gluten antigen presentation.[24]

HLA-DQ2.5 has a positively charged peptide-binding groove, which preferentially binds peptides with negatively charged amino acids at anchor positions P4, P6, and P7.[25] Proline-rich (P), glutamine-rich (Q) gliadin peptides (Q-X-P sequence) that survived GI digestion are excellent substrates for TTG and can selectively be deamidated, resulting in peptides that are negatively charged due to the presence of multiple glutamic acid residues. These prolin-rich, deamidated gliadin peptides are highly immunogenic due to their increased avidity and superior binding to the positively charged groove of HLA-DQ2.5. Similarly, HLA-DQ8 also has positively charged binding groove, preferentially binding to negatively charged residues at anchor positions P1, P4, and P9.[26] Proline residues in gliadin peptides not only confer particular resistance to proteolysis by digestive enzymes but naturally adopt a left-handed polyproline II helical conformation, which is the preferred conformation of all bound HLA Class II ligands, such as the PQPQLPY motif frequently found in immunodominant α-gliadin epitopes.

Presentation of gliadin peptides to T cells through HLA-DQ2 or DQ8 will result in selective gluten-specific CD4+ T cell activation and clonal expansion in the intestinal mucosa of patients with CD[27] **(Fig. 2)**. Activated CD4+ T cells produce Th1 cytokines, including tumor necrosis factor alpha, interferon gamma, IL-18, and IL-21. In addition, IL-15 produced by gluten-exposed epithelial cells also contributes to the proinflammatory environment. The concerted effect of the proinflammatory cytokines will activate cytotoxic CD8+ T cells and natural killer (NK) cells. In addition, Th2 cytokines produced by gluten-specific CD4+ T cells provide help to B cells to differentiate into antibody-secreting plasma cells, which will produce antibodies to deamidated gliadin peptides (DGP) and TTG. Eventually, concerted effector functions including activated cytotoxic CD8+ T cells and NK cells, as well as anti-TTG antibody-mediated responses, result in destruction of mucosal epithelial cells.[28] The mucosal damage evolves into villous atrophy characteristic of CD, with significant lymphocytic infiltrates and epithelial hyperplasia.[10]

LABORATORY DIAGNOSTICS OF CELIAC DISEASE
Serologic Testing

For most patients with suspicion of CD, serology testing is an important part of the diagnostic workup. Given that gluten is the inciting antigen, it would make sense to

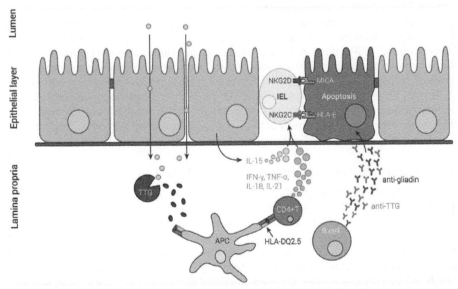

Fig. 2. Overview of the immune response to gluten peptides in celiac disease. Tissue transglutaminase (TTG) deamidates gliadin peptides derived from gluten, which are then processed by dendritic cells and presented through HLA-DQ2.5 and DQ8 molecules to CD4+ T cells. Activated gluten reactive CD4+ T cells will then produce Th1 cytokines including tumor necrosis factor alpha, interferon gamma, IL-18, and IL-21. IL-15 secreted by intestinal epithelial cells in response to gluten also contributes to the proinflammatory environment. The proinflammatory cytokine milieu will induce activation of intraepithelial lymphocytes (IEL) leading to apoptosis and increased intestinal permeability. CD4+ T cells will also provide help to B cells and induce differentiation into plasma cells, which will produce antibodies to DGP and TTG. Activation of these T cell– and antibody-mediated mechanisms results in villous atrophy typical of celiac disease pathology.

predict that patients with CD might develop antibodies against this protein. Gluten, the principal component of wheat protein (90%) is a complex consistent of gliadin and glutenin. It is actually gliadin that triggers the immune response in CD, because of several unique properties that make it particularly immunogenic, as discussed earlier. Presentation of the immunogenic gliadin peptide by HLA-DQ2.5 or DQ8 can lead to T-cell activation and ultimately the development of an antigen-specific antibody response.

One of the first serologic markers for CD was antigliadin antibodies. Although used diagnostically for years, this test had significant limitations such as low specificity. Because immune reactivity against DGP has been shown to be more prominent compared with the native peptide,[29,30] the possibility of using these modified peptides as more specific epitopes for antibody detection emerged.[31] Eventually, detection of antibodies against the deamidated form of gliadin had much improved diagnostic utility. In some of the first studies comparing the 2 markers, antibodies to partially deamidated gliadin peptides had a sensitivity and specificity of 92% and 90%, respectively, compared with 87% and 72% for antibodies against unmodified gliadin.[32] At this time, testing for antigliadin antibodies has largely been phased out of the clinical laboratory, having been replaced by DGP antibody.

Another early serologic marker of CD was the endomysial antibody (EMA). EMA was so named because it was observed that patients with CD had antibodies that bound to the connective tissue surrounding smooth muscle fibers.[33] This connective tissue is known as the endomysium. EMA became a diagnostic test for CD, largely based on very high specificities, approaching 100% in some studies.[34–36] Currently, EMA testing is generally available from most large reference laboratories, still being performed by the indirect immunofluorescence (IIF) methodology. Although reagents for EMA testing are commercially available, the expertise required for reading and interpretation of the slides has precluded its widespread implementation.

Because of the challenges associated with IIF for EMA, it was desirable to convert this testing to a more high-throughput method, such as enzyme immunoassay (EIA). However, this would require knowledge of the specific antigen within the endomysium to which the EMA was binding. This antigen was eventually identified, and it turned out to be the enzyme TTG—the same enzyme responsible for the deamidation of the gliadin peptides in the lamina propria region of the small intestine, which confers the pathogenic potential to these peptides.[37] Original diagnostic studies of tests for anti-TTG antibodies were encouraging. Although most studies concluded that the specificity of anti-TTG antibody was slightly lower than EMA, it was still well greater than 90% to 95%. In addition, reported sensitivities of anti-TTG antibodies were apparently higher than that of EMA, also in the range of 90% to 95%,[34] which led to rapid development and Food and Drug Administration (FDA) approval of a variety of assays for anti-TTG antibodies. Based on a review of the College of American Pathologists proficiency testing survey, there are more than 20 commercially available anti-TTG antibody assays being used in clinical laboratories across the United States. Originally, most assays were developed as EIAs, although this is now expanding with bead-based multiplex immunoassays and electrochemiluminescent assays also being available.

Despite the advances and improvements in serologic testing, there are some important limitations. One limitation is related to the primary treatment for CD, specifically the GFD. The goal of the GFD is to remove the antigenic stimulation from the immune system, thereby leading to attenuation and eventually quiescence of the inflammatory response. Most patients respond quite well to this treatment, showing clinical remission and resolution of symptoms. The consequence of this treatment is a decline in celiac-specific antibody production, which is useful for physicians monitoring patients for their response to the GFD: a decrease in antibody levels is an indication that the gluten has successfully been removed from the patient's diet. However, this is a limitation of testing that can complicate the diagnosis, because if the patient is on GFD at the time of diagnosis, the result may be a false-negative result. Awareness of CD is increasing in the general population and so is exposure to gluten-free foods. An individual with GI or other symptoms might preemptively start a GFD before presenting to their physician. In this context, the value of serologic testing is questionable. If the patient has CD, a positive result is possible, depending on the extent and duration of which gluten has been eliminated. On the other hand, a negative result does not exclude CD, because it may well be the consequence of the GFD. In this case, further workup might be necessary, including a gluten challenge. Although this might be a less-than-attractive option to the patient, it may be the only way to overcome the interference of the GFD on the serologic testing.

A second limitation of serologic testing is related to the isotype of the EMA, TTG, and DGP antibodies. Although, at least for TTG and DGP antibodies, IgA and IgG isotypes are routinely available, the IgA isotypes tend to have the highest sensitivity and specificity. This is especially true for anti-TTG antibodies. The complicating factor to this is a condition referred to as selective IgA deficiency. Selective IgA deficiency is an absence of IgA production in the context of normal IgG and IgM concentrations. Patients with selective IgA deficiency generally do not show signs of immunodeficiency. However, it tends to be more common in patients with CD. The absence of IgA production precludes the use of TTG-IgA, EMA-IgA, and DPG-IgA antibodies for the diagnostic evaluation of CD due to the risk of a false-negative result. For these patients, testing for the IgG isotype is necessary. It is for this reason that total IgA testing is recommended as part of the diagnostic evaluation of suspected CD; it allows for identification of patients with selective IgA deficiency and can direct appropriate celiac-specific serology testing.

In addition to serology testing (**Table 1**), endoscopy is routinely used for the diagnosis of CD. Endoscopy is an invasive procedure in which a flexible tube is passed through the esophagus and stomach, and into the small intestine. At the front end of the tube is camera, which allows the physician to visualize the gross anatomy of the small intestine. Instruments at the end of the tube can also be used to extract pieces of tissue for histologic evaluation. For CD, biopsy histology is the most important part of the endoscopy, compared with visualization of the gross anatomy. Some features of the biopsy that would be consistent with CD include atrophy of the small intestinal villi (shortening of the fingerlike projections that absorb nutrients from digested food), crypt hyperplasia (thickening of grooves between the villi), and intraepithelial lymphocytosis (increased numbers of lymphocytes within the GI mucosa). Although these features, particularly the atrophy and crypt hyperplasia, suggest CD, they are not diagnostic. In fact, these abnormalities can be seen in other conditions, including tropical sprue, bacterial overgrowth, and chronic variable immunodeficiency. On the other hand, it is possible to find a normal biopsy in a patient with active CD. Sometimes the areas of villous atrophy are "patchy"; a normal or abnormal interpretation could be obtained, depending on where the biopsy is sampled from. It is for this reason that it is recommended to obtain a minimum of 4 tissue pieces from different areas of the small intestine, including the duodenal bulb. Sample quality is also critical, and is related to the tissue processing and orientation. For example, if the biopsy specimen is oriented suboptimally, the villi/crypt ratio could be underestimated, leading to a falsely abnormal interpretation. Given these limitations, it is not advised to establish a diagnosis of CD based on biopsy alone; correlation with celiac-specific serologies is optimal.

Several professional organizations have published recommendations related to the diagnosis of CD. Most guidelines include suggestions of which patients should be tested and how. In some cases, the guidelines divided these patient groups into "high" and "low" pretest probability categories, with different testing options for each. For example, both the American College of Gastroenterology (ACG) and the World Gastroenterology Organization (WGO) suggest that patients with a high pretest probability of CD should have anti-TTG-IgA testing and a small intestinal biopsy.[38,39] In comparison, patients with low pretest probabilities should be screened serologically first and only have endoscopy if the serology result is positive. Also, the ACG and WGO guidelines deal with the issue of IgA deficiency, although in different ways. In patients for whom the diagnosis of CD is less certain, the ACG recommends total IgA in addition to anti-TTG-IgA, whereas the WGO suggests the use of anti-DGP-IgG along with anti-TTG-IgA. Another group, the European Society for Pediatric Gastroenterology, Hepatology, and Nutrition (ESPGHAN), has published guidelines for the diagnosis of CD in children.[40] These recommendations differ from the ACG and WGO in 2 significant ways. First, the ESPGHAN recommendations rely on HLA typing more significantly. For example, the ESPGHAN suggests that HLA typing be the initial test in high-risk patients who are asymptomatic, with follow-up testing using total IgA and anti-TTG-IgA for patients who carry the genetic risk factor. Second, these guidelines indicate that it may be possible to make a diagnosis of CD in the absence of a biopsy. For symptomatic children, testing would begin with total IgA and anti-TTG-IgA. If the anti-TTG-IgA result is positive but less than 10-fold greater than the upper limit of normal (ULN), a biopsy is recommended. However, if the anti-TTG-IgA result is more than 10-fold greater than the ULN, then ESPGHAN suggests that CD could be confirmed by EMA and HLA typing. Although it must be highlighted that these different guidelines were prepared with different patient populations in mind, it is clear that there is still no total agreement on the best testing approach for the diagnosis of CD.

HLA Testing

HLA testing for HLA-DQ2 and DQ8 is clinically available and routinely performed in many laboratories. It is important to highlight that while the presence of HLA-DQ2 or DQ8 is necessary to develop CD, the presence of either one of them is not diagnostic for CD because it has a very low positive predictive value. The absence of HLA-DQ2 and DQ8 however virtually rules out the diagnosis of CD, because it has a negative predictive value greater than 99%.

Guidelines for diagnosis of CD from the ESPGHAN proposed for the first time the option to omit duodenal biopsy for the diagnosis of CD in children and adolescents, if (1) clinical signs and symptoms that suggest CD are present, (2) anti-TTG antibody level is increased more than 10 times the upper limit of normal, (3) confirmatory EMA antibody from a second sample is positive, and (4) the patient expresses the HLA-DQ2 or DQ8 risk alleles.[40] For asymptomatic children and adolescents with CD-associated conditions the recommendation is to offer HLA testing as a first-line test, because the absence of HLA DQ2 or DQ8 renders CD highly unlikely, and no further follow-up with serologic tests is necessary.

Because the chance of an individual negative for HLA-DQ2 or HLA-DQ8 having CD is extremely small, the main role of HLA-DQ typing in the diagnosis of CD is to exclude the disease. Clinical indications include equivocal small bowel histologic findings in seronegative individuals, or discrepancies between serology and histology, or evaluation of individuals not tested for CD before starting a GFD, or the presence of strong serologic and clinical evidence when biopsy is not possible or preferred (eg, children).

Table 1
Testing options available for diagnostic evaluation of suspected celiac disease

Test	Analyte/Target	Methodology	Clinical Utility			Affected by	
			Initial Diagnostic Test	Secondary Diagnostic Test	Monitoring Response to Gluten-free Diet	Selective IgA Deficiency	Gluten-Free Diet
Total IgA	Immunoglobulin IgA	Nephelometry	Yes	Yes	No	Yes	No
Gliadin IgA	Native gliadin	Antigen-specific immunoassay	No	No	No	Yes	Yes
Gliadin IgG			No	No	No	No	Yes
EMA IgA	TTG	Indirect immunofluorescence	No	Yes	No	Yes	Yes
TTG IgA		Antigen-specific immunoassay	Yes	Yes	Yes	Yes	Yes
TTG IgG			No	Yes	Yes	No	Yes
DGP IgA	Deamidated gliadin peptides	Antigen-specific immunoassay	No	Yes	Yes	Yes	Yes
DGP IgG			Maybe	Yes	Yes	No	Yes
Biopsy	Inflammation and damage in small intestine	Endoscopy and biopsy with evaluation for villous atrophy, crypt hyperplasia, and IEL enumeration	Maybe	Yes	Maybe	No	Yes
HLA-DQ2/DQ8	Genetic risk factor	HLA typing, detection of HLA-DQ2 and HLA-DQ8	No	Yes	No	No	No

In addition, HLA typing plays important role in ruling out individuals who belong to groups at risk for CD, such as first-degree relatives of patients with confirmed CD or conditions known to be associated with CD such as autoimmune diseases including T1D, liver, and thyroid disease; chromosomal abnormalities including Williams, Turner, and Down syndromes; and selective IgA deficiency.[40]

Methodologies that are commonly used include genotyping by sequence-specific oligonucleotide probe (SSOP) hybridization, which is currently the FDA-cleared gold standard in HLA laboratories. The SSOP method provides information on gene dose and allele copy number, which provides additional risk assessment option to clinicians. Method limitations for SSOP include ambiguities due to probing for exon 2 only as opposed to the full-length DQB1 gene. The result is reported out with an allele code and a string of alleles, the order of which reflects their frequencies in the population, common and well-documented alleles being shown as preferred choice in the string.

In addition to SSOP, laboratory-developed real-time PCR followed by melting curve analysis is also used as a fast and cost-effective alternative.[41] This method provides qualitative, positive or negative result for each allele tested and does not provide information on allele copy numbers. Limitations of traditional methodologies can be eliminated by sequencing of the entire length of the HLA genes, using Next Generation Sequencing (NGS)–based HLA genotyping, an emerging methodology currently conquering the HLA typing field across clinical laboratories. NGS is able to provide unambiguous allele level results and information on the number of alleles present. Limitations include complexity and cost, which can be mitigated by batching a larger number of samples, making it a viable approach for clinical laboratories.

SUMMARY

Two thousand years after the first description of CD, the understanding of the disease is finally converging toward a mechanistic appreciation of pathogenesis, in which HLA-DQ2 and DQ8 orchestrate the immune response to gluten peptides, resulting in the specific intestinal pathology. However, not everybody expressing HLA-DQ2 or DQ8 and exposed to gluten develops CD, suggesting that much more work is needed to elucidate the additional genetic and environmental factors that control the onset of CD development.

Because of variable penetrance and highly variable presentation the diagnosis of CD can be challenging, and the disease is often underdiagnosed. Identification of the gluten-induced mechanism allowed for the study of gluten-specific immune response and definition of antigenic targets, such as DGP and TTG. Antibodies against these molecules can be detected in patients with CD, representing important diagnostic tools. Diagnostic guidelines have been developed by regulatory organizations, showing heterogeneity in testing algorithms, targeting different patient populations. Intestinal biopsies still constitute the gold standard for diagnosis. Genetic testing for HLA-DQ2 and DQ8 is not diagnostic, because the frequencies of these alleles are much higher in the population compared with the incidence of CD, but it is very useful for ruling out disease, because the absence of HLA-DQ2.5 or DQ8 will practically exclude CD. Recent guidelines from the ESPGHAN place greater emphasis on HLA testing, which can be used as a first-line test in select pediatric patients with CD-specific signs and symptoms, and persistent high-level antibodies, when biopsy is not an option or is not desired. Despite significant developments in CD diagnostics, therapeutic approaches are still lagging behind. Sixty-five years after the discovery of the efficacy of GFD as the treatment for CD, this therapy is still the gold-standard treatment for CD. Approaches targeting the gluten-specific immune response, TTG inhibitors, or proteases targeting immunogenic peptides in the intestinal lumen are under investigation and may open new therapeutic opportunities in the future. Recently, a Phase I clinical trial was completed using epitope-specific CD4+ immunotherapy with the goal of rendering gluten-specific T cells unresponsive to further antigenic stimulation,[42] indicating the possibility of vaccines becoming part of CD therapy in the future.

ACKNOWLEDGMENTS

The authors acknowledge the expert help of Mary Paul and Natalya Wilkins-Tyler in preparation of the figures.

REFERENCES

1. Gasbarrini G, Rickards O, Martinez-Labarga C, et al. Origin of celiac disease: how old are predisposing haplotypes? World J Gastroenterol 2012;18(37):5300–4.
2. Van De Kamer JH, Weijers HA, Dicke WK. Coeliac disease. IV. An investigation into the injurious constituents of wheat in connection with their action on patients with coeliac disease. Acta Paediatr 1953;42(3):223–31.
3. Seah PP, Fry L, Rossiter MA, et al. Anti-reticulin antibodies in childhood coeliac disease. Lancet 1971;2(7726):681–2.
4. Bevan S, Popat S, Braegger CP, et al. Contribution of the MHC region to the familial risk of coeliac disease. J Med Genet 1999;36(9):687–90.
5. Sollid LM, Markussen G, Ek J, et al. Evidence for a primary association of celiac disease to a particular HLA-DQ alpha/beta heterodimer. J Exp Med 1989;169(1): 345–50.
6. Sollid LM. Coeliac disease: dissecting a complex inflammatory disorder. Nat Rev Immunol 2002;2(9):647–55.
7. Concannon P, Rich SS, Nepom GT. Genetics of type 1A diabetes. N Engl J Med 2009;360(16):1646–54.
8. Karell K, Louka AS, Moodie SJ, et al. HLA types in celiac disease patients not carrying the DQA1*05-DQB1*02 (DQ2) heterodimer: results from the European Genetics Cluster on Celiac Disease. Hum Immunol 2003;64(4):469–77.
9. Bodd M, Kim CY, Lundin KE, et al. T-cell response to gluten in patients with HLA-DQ2.2 reveals requirement of peptide-MHC stability in celiac disease. Gastroenterology 2012;142(3):552–61.
10. Gujral N, Freeman HJ, Thomson AB. Celiac disease: prevalence, diagnosis, pathogenesis and treatment. World J Gastroenterol 2012;18(42):6036–59.
11. Fasano A, Berti I, Gerarduzzi T, et al. Prevalence of celiac disease in at-risk and not-at-risk groups in the United States: a large multicenter study. Arch Intern Med 2003;163(3):286–92.
12. Meresse B, Malamut G, Cerf-Bensussan N. Celiac disease: an immunological jigsaw. Immunity 2012;36(6):907–19.
13. Margaritte-Jeannin P, Babron MC, Bourgey M, et al. HLA-DQ relative risks for coeliac disease in European populations: a study of the European Genetics Cluster on Coeliac Disease. Tissue Antigens 2004;63(6):562–7.
14. Ploski R, Ek J, Thorsby E, et al. On the HLA-DQ(alpha 1*0501, beta 1*0201)-associated susceptibility in celiac disease: a possible gene dosage effect of DQB1*0201. Tissue Antigens 1993;41(4):173–7.

15. Vader W, Stepniak D, Kooy Y, et al. The HLA-DQ2 gene dose effect in celiac disease is directly related to the magnitude and breadth of gluten-specific T cell responses. Proc Natl Acad Sci U S A 2003;100(21):12390–5.

16. Pietzak MM, Schofield TC, McGinniss MJ, et al. Stratifying risk for celiac disease in a large at-risk United States population by using HLA alleles. Clin Gastroenterol Hepatol 2009;7(9):966–71.

17. Liu E, Lee HS, Aronsson CA, et al. Risk of pediatric celiac disease according to HLA haplotype and country. N Engl J Med 2014;371(1):42–9.

18. van Heel DA, Franke L, Hunt KA, et al. A genome-wide association study for celiac disease identifies risk variants in the region harboring IL2 and IL21. Nat Genet 2007;39(7):827–9.

19. Horton R, Wilming L, Rand V, et al. Gene map of the extended human MHC. Nat Rev Genet 2004;5(12):889–99.

20. Nistico L, Fagnani C, Coto I, et al. Concordance, disease progression, and heritability of coeliac disease in Italian twins. Gut 2006;55(6):803–8.

21. Trynka G, Hunt KA, Bockett NA, et al. Dense genotyping identifies and localizes multiple common and rare variant association signals in celiac disease. Nat Genet 2011;43(12):1193–201.

22. Withoff S, Li Y, Jonkers I, et al. Understanding celiac disease by genomics. Trends Genet 2016;32(5):295–308.

23. Kumar V, Wijmenga C, Withoff S. From genome-wide association studies to disease mechanisms: celiac disease as a model for autoimmune diseases. Semin Immunopathol 2012;34(4):567–80.

24. Fallang LE, Bergseng E, Hotta K, et al. Differences in the risk of celiac disease associated with HLA-DQ2.5 or HLA-DQ2.2 are related to sustained gluten antigen presentation. Nat Immunol 2009;10(10):1096–101.

25. Jones EY, Fugger L, Strominger JL, et al. MHC class II proteins and disease: a structural perspective. Nat Rev Immunol 2006;6(4):271–82.

26. Abadie V, Sollid LM, Barreiro LB, et al. Integration of genetic and immunological insights into a model of celiac disease pathogenesis. Annu Rev Immunol 2011; 29:493–525.

27. Lundin KE, Scott H, Hansen T, et al. Gliadin-specific, HLA-DQ(alpha 1*0501,beta 1*0201) restricted T cells isolated from the small intestinal mucosa of celiac disease patients. J Exp Med 1993;178(1):187–96.

28. Di Sabatino A, Corazza GR. Coeliac disease. Lancet 2009;373(9673):1480–93.

29. Molberg O, McAdam SN, Korner R, et al. Tissue transglutaminase selectively modifies gliadin peptides that are recognized by gut-derived T cells in celiac disease. Nat Med 1998;4(6):713–7.

30. Sjostrom H, Lundin KE, Molberg O, et al. Identification of a gliadin T-cell epitope in coeliac disease: general importance of gliadin deamidation for intestinal T-cell recognition. Scand J Immunol 1998;48(2):111–5.

31. Aleanzi M, Demonte AM, Esper C, et al. Celiac disease: antibody recognition against native and selectively deamidated gliadin peptides. Clin Chem 2001; 47(11):2023–8.

32. Ankelo M, Kleimola V, Simell S, et al. Antibody responses to deamidated gliadin peptide show high specificity and parallel antibodies to tissue transglutaminase in developing coeliac disease. Clin Exp Immunol 2007;150(2):285–93.

33. Chorzelski TP, Beutner EH, Sulej J, et al. IgA anti-endomysium antibody. A new immunological marker of dermatitis herpetiformis and coeliac disease. Br J Dermatol 1984;111(4):395–402.

34. Giersiepen K, Lelgemann M, Stuhldreher N, et al. Accuracy of diagnostic anti-body tests for coeliac disease in children: summary of an evidence report. J Pediatr Gastroenterol Nutr 2012;54(2):229–41.
35. Kurppa K, Rasanen T, Collin P, et al. Endomysial antibodies predict celiac disease irrespective of the titers or clinical presentation. World J Gastroenterol 2012;18(20):2511–6.
36. Ferreira M, Davies SL, Butler M, et al. Endomysial antibody: is it the best screening test for coeliac disease? Gut 1992;33(12):1633–7.
37. Dieterich W, Ehnis T, Bauer M, et al. Identification of tissue transglutaminase as the autoantigen of celiac disease. Nat Med 1997;3(7):797–801.
38. World gastroenterology organisation global guidelines - celiac disease. World Gastroenterology Organisation; 2016. Available at: http://www.worldgastroenterology.org/UserFiles/file/guidelines/celiac-disease-english-2016.pdf. Accessed July 3, 2018.
39. Rubio-Tapia A, Hill ID, Kelly CP, et al. ACG clinical guidelines: diagnosis and management of celiac disease. Am J Gastroenterol 2013;108(5):656–76 [quiz: 677].
40. Husby S, Koletzko S, Korponay-Szabo IR, et al. European Society for Pediatric Gastroenterology, Hepatology, and Nutrition guidelines for the diagnosis of coeliac disease. J Pediatr Gastroenterol Nutr 2012;54(1):136–60.
41. Profaizer T, Eckels D, Delgado JC. Celiac disease and HLA typing using real-time PCR with melting curve analysis. Tissue Antigens 2011;78(1):31–7.
42. Goel G, King T, Daveson AJ, et al. Epitope-specific immunotherapy targeting CD4-positive T cells in coeliac disease: two randomised, double-blind, placebo-controlled phase 1 studies. Lancet Gastroenterol Hepatol 2017;2(7):479–93.

Human Leukocyte Antigen Associations in Drug Hypersensitivity Reactions

Ryan J. Schutte, PhD[a], Yonghu Sun, MD, PhD[b], Danmeng Li, MD[a], Furen Zhang, MD, PhD[b], David A. Ostrov, PhD[a],*

KEYWORDS

- HLA • HLA associated • Hypersensitivity • Adverse drug reactions • ADRs
- Abacavir • Dapsone • Prediction

KEY POINTS

- Specific HLA alleles have been strongly associated with well-characterized drug hypersensitivities.
- Multiple mechanisms likely mediate HLA-associated drug hypersensitivities.
- The disparity between negative and positive predictive values limits mechanism characterization.
- Prediction of hypersensitivity may be improved by including other HLA variants and risk-associated biomarkers in pharmacogenetic testing.

INTRODUCTION

Traditionally, drug hypersensitivity syndromes that are T-cell mediated have been classified as Gell and Coombs type IV reactions. This classification has recently been updated to include 4 subtypes to represent key effector cell populations involved in the reaction (IVa macrophage, IVb eosinophil, IVc T cell, and IVd neutrophil).[1] The syndromes include drug-induced hypersensitivity syndrome, drug reaction with eosinophilia, hypersensitivity syndrome, Stevens-Johnson syndrome/toxic epidermal necrolysis (SJS/TEN), acute generalized exanthematous pustulosis, drug-induced lupus, fixed drug eruption, and single-organ involvement pathologies such as drug-induced

Disclosure Statement: The authors have no relationships with a commercial company that has a direct financial interest in subject matter or materials discussed in article or with a company making a competing product.
Funding: This work was funded by NIH NIAID R01 AI103348.
[a] Department of Pathology, Immunology and Laboratory Medicine, University of Florida College of Medicine, University of Florida, PO Box 103633, Gainesville, FL 32610-3633, USA;
[b] Department of Dermatology, Shandong Provincial Institute of Dermatology and Venereology, 27397 Jingshi Road, Jinan, Shandong 250022, PR China
* Corresponding author.
E-mail address: ostroda@pathology.ufl.edu

Clin Lab Med 38 (2018) 669–677
https://doi.org/10.1016/j.cll.2018.08.002
0272-2712/18/© 2018 Elsevier Inc. All rights reserved.

labmed.theclinics.com

liver disease (DILI). These syndromes are considered immunologically mediated, although toxic mechanisms may be important contributing factors for DILI.

HLA alleles have been strongly associated with well-characterized drug hypersensitivities (Table 1),[2–4] including HLA-B*57:01 with abacavir hypersensitivity syndrome,[5,6] HLA-B*15:02 with carbamazepine-induced SJS/TEN in Asian populations,[7,8] HLA-B*58:01 with allopurinol-induced hypersensitivity syndrome,[9] and HLA-B*13:01 with dapsone hypersensitivity syndrome.[10] The associations between specific HLA alleles and hypersensitivities in response to abacavir, carbamazepine, and allopurinol were extraordinarily strong (odds ratios >800, see Table 1).

MULTIPLE MECHANISMS OF IMMUNE RECOGNITION MEDIATE HLA-ASSOCIATED DRUG HYPERSENSITIVITY

Because the main function of classic polymorphic HLA molecules is to present peptides for recognition by T cells, genetic associations between drug hypersensitivity and specific HLA implicate mechanisms involving binding interactions between drugs, HLA molecules and, potentially, T-cell antigen receptors (TCR).

Drugs may modify the HLA-dependent TCR interface by one or several described mechanisms (Fig. 1). The hapten (or prohapten) mechanism describes drugs and their metabolites that form adducts with self-proteins in the host that lead to immune recognition of the resulting hapten:self-peptide complexes as de novo antigens (see Fig. 1).[11] The pharmacologic interaction mechanism (pi model) describes drugs that noncovalently and reversibly bind HLA (and or TCR) molecules without binding the antigen-binding cleft.[12] The altered repertoire model is a mechanism in which a drug binds within the antigen-binding cleft of associated HLA molecules.[13] In this latter model, the drug alters the repertoire of HLA-bound peptides, resulting in the presentation of self-peptides to which the host has not been tolerized.

The altered repertoire mechanism is consistent with data showing direct intramolecular interactions between abacavir, peptide, and HLA-B*57:01, which was strongly

Table 1
Specific HLA alleles have been strongly associated with drug hypersensitivities

Drug and Syndrome	HLA Allele	HLA Carriage Rate	Disease Prevalence	OR	NPV	PPV
Abacavir DHR	B*57:01	5%–8% Caucasian	8%	960	100% for patch test confirmed	55%
Allopurinol SJS/TEN and DRESS/DIHS	B*58:01	9%–20% Han Chinese; 1%–6% Caucasian	0.1%–0.4%	>800	100% in Han Chinese	3%
Carbamazepine SJS/TEN	B*15:02	10%–15% Han Chinese; <0.1% Caucasian	<0.1%–0.6%	>1000	100% in Han Chinese	3%
Dapsone DRESS/ DIHS	B*13:01	2%–20% Han Chinese	1%–4% Han Chinese	20	99.8%	7.8%[10]

However, not all subjects carrying the associated HLA allele will develop drug hypersensitivity (eg, 3% for allopurinol).

Abbreviations: DHR, drug hypersensitivity reaction; DIHS, drug-induced hypersensitivity syndrome; DRESS, drug reaction with eosinophilia; NPV, negative predictive value; OR, odds ratio; PPV, positive predictive value.

Data from White KD, Abe R, Ardern-Jones M, et al. SJS/TEN 2017: building multidisciplinary networks to drive science and translation. J Allergy Clin Immunol Pract 2018;6(1):38–69.

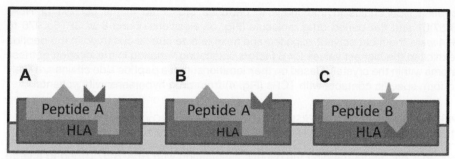

Fig. 1. HLA-associated drug hypersensitivity reactions may be mediated by at least 3 binding mechanisms: (*A*) small molecule drugs or their metabolites may act as haptens, forming adducts with peptides presented by HLA molecules, (*B*) drugs may form direct noncovalent interactions with solvent accessible portions of associated HLA molecules (and/or TCRs), and (*C*) drugs may bind within the antigen-binding cleft, altering the repertoire of HLA-bound peptides and permitting presentation of self-peptides to which the host has not been tolerized.

associated with a systemic hypersensitivity syndrome. Three independent groups showed that abacavir altered the repertoire of peptides bound to HLA-B*57:01.[13–15] Structures of HLA-B*57:01 complexed with abacavir and synthetic peptides were determined by X-ray crystallography. The structures showed that the drug formed noncovalent interactions with peptide and amino acids in the antigen-binding cleft of HLA-B*57:01.[13,15] A self-peptide recognized by T cells from abacavir hypersensitivity patients (VTTDIQVKV, corresponding to the human early transcription elongation factor of RNA pol II elongation factor SPT5a, residues 976–984) was defined by eluting peptides from abacavir-treated cells expressing HLA-B*57:01 and testing peptides for recognition by T cells from abacavir hypersensitivity patients.

The crystal structure of abacavir complexed to self-peptide SPT5a 976 to 984 and HLA-B*57:01 (**Fig. 2**)[16] revealed that T cells were unlikely to have direct binding specificity for the drug abacavir because it is buried in the antigen-binding cleft and not solvent accessible. Instead, T cells presumably formed specific contacts with exposed

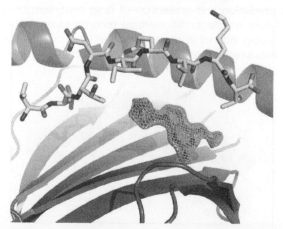

Fig. 2. The crystal structure of an immunogenic self-peptide complexed to abacavir and HLA-B*57:01 revealed solvent accessible side chains available for recognition by T cells. Abacavir is shown as cyan chicken wire in an omit electron density map in the top panel.

peptide side chains in immunogenic peptides presented in the context of HLA-B*57:01 and the buried drug molecule (**Fig. 3**). Positions 4 and 8 of SPT5a 976 to 984 were the most solvent-exposed and flexible side chains observed in the peptide (exhibited the highest values for B factors, indicating variation in the location of these atoms within the crystal). Based on their locations, these peptide side chains are likely to form specific contacts with TCRs (**Fig. 4**) from drug hypersensitivity patients.

PREDICTION OF DRUG HYPERSENSITIVITY MAY BE IMPROVED BY COMBINING RISK-ASSOCIATED BIOMARKERS WITH RISK-ASSOCIATED HLA ALLELES

For abacavir, understanding the genetic association with HLA-B*57:01 led to a large double-blind, prospective, randomized study showing that exclusion from abacavir treatment based on a pharmacogenetic test successfully prevented abacavir hypersensitivity syndrome.[17] The Food and Drug Administration (FDA) consequently instituted a Boxed Warning about the recommendation to test all patients for the HLA-B*57:01 allele before starting or restarting therapy with abacavir or abacavir-containing medications.[18] Although the association between HLA-B*57:01 and abacavir is sufficient to predict at-risk patients in a cost-effective manner, HLA alleles associated with drug hypersensitivities are limited in their utility, in part, because of low positive predictive value (PPV, true positives/true positives + false positives). An idealized prediction test would exhibit 100% PPV and 100% negative predictive value (NPV, true negatives/true negatives + false negatives). For the well-characterized drug hypersensitivities shown in **Table 1**, HLA alleles were associated with nearly 100% NPV, but PPV ranged from 3% to 55%.[19] These data indicate that specific HLA alleles are necessary for specific drug hypersensitivities but are not sufficient to mediate the adverse responses without other genetic or environmental factors.

These data illustrate a significant limitation to prediction of drug hypersensitivity by testing for single HLA alleles. Drug hypersensitivity reactions occur exclusively in individuals carrying specific HLA types, but only a critical, unpredictable subset of these individuals will develop the adverse drug reactions (ADRs) (3% for allopurinol-induced SJS/TEN).[19] The gap between negative and positive predictive values is a significant limitation in understanding immunopathologic mechanisms and in the prediction of risk for drug hypersensitivity reactions.

More accurate prediction and prevention of drug hypersensitivities will likely be achieved in the future as electronic medical records incorporate whole genome sequencing, HLA typing, and other biomarkers that have been associated with drug hypersensitivity (discussed later). Because HLA-associated drug hypersensitivities

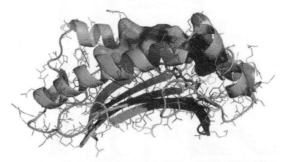

Fig. 3. The crystal structure of self peptide VTTDIQVKV SPT5a 976 to 984 complexed to abacavir and HLA-B*57:01 is shown with the peptide colored by B factor with red indicating the highest degree of flexibility.

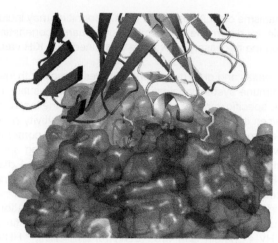

Fig. 4. An HLA-B–restricted TCR (*gray lines*), from PDB code 2NX5, was superimposed to display the location of putative TCR contact sites, with respect to a conventional TCR docking mode.

are dependent on additional genetic and environmental factors, the risk of an individual developing a drug hypersensitivity reaction will likely be refined by algorithms that account for associated HLA alleles, other genetic variants, viral infection, and possibly markers of inflammation or other biomarkers yet to be discovered.

There are several types of genetic variants that may be considered as potential drug hypersensitivity biomarkers in association with specific HLA alleles. Genes encoding proteins involved in drug metabolism have been associated with ADRs. Genes relevant to drug hypersensitivity that have been shown to influence drug metabolism include P450 genes such as CYP34A[20] and CYP2C9,[21] myeloperoxidase,[22] glutamate-cysteine ligase catalytic subunit gene GCLC,[23] and mitochondrial antidefense pathway Nrf-2.[24] Effects of other well-characterized polymorphic genes involved in metabolism on risk of HLA-associated drug hypersensitivity (such as CYP2D6, CYP2C19, N-acetyl transferase, thiopurine methyltransferase) are not known but may influence risk by altering the concentration of drug/metabolite[25] available for recognition by HLA-restricted T cells. Variants that influence drug absorption, distribution, metabolism, and excretion (ADME) may similarly influence risk of HLA-associated hypersensitivity. A consensus core list of 184 ADME predictors of pharmacokinetic variability that could affect drug safety and efficacy in the current drug development was defined for pharmaceutical clinical trials and FDA drug submissions. Analysis of ADME predictors in the context of patients expressing HLA alleles associated with high levels of risk drug hypersensitivity may improve positive predictive values of pharmacogenetics tests.

Drug hypersensitivities strongly associated with class I HLA alleles suggest that immunopathologic mechanisms involve recognition by TCRs of CD8$^+$ T cells or by natural killer (NK) cells. Killer immunoglobulin-like receptors (KIR) are highly polymorphic receptors expressed on NK cells that have been shown to interact with class I HLA molecules. Their roles in drug hypersensitivity have been hypothesized[26] but not well studied. The 16 most polymorphic KIR genes are 2DL1, 2DL2, 2DL3, 2DL4, 2DL5, 2DS1, 2DS2, 2DS3, 2DS4, 2DS5, 3DL1, 3DS1, 3DL2, 3DL3, 2DP1, and 3DP1. Because specific HLA alleles associated with drug hypersensitivity have been shown to be KIR ligands (eg, HLA-B*57:01 and HLA-B*58:01, HLA-Bw4 ligands for 3DL1[27]), mechanisms of HLA-restricted drug recognition may include KIR binding. It will be possible to determine if specificity of pharmacogenetic tests may be improved based on the necessary HLA allele combined with KIR variants associated with risk.

Autoimmune diseases and drug hypersensitivity responses both involve stimulation of the adaptive immune system against self-proteins and tissues. Therefore, pleiotropic and disease-specific variants in confirmed autoimmune loci would be expected to be observed when comparing populations of hypersensitivity patients with drug-tolerant patients expressing the same HLA allele. There are confirmed autoimmune loci associated with seronegative (psoriasis 36 loci, ankylosing spondylitis 31) and seropositive autoimmune diseases (celiac disease 40 loci, type 1 diabetes 43, rheumatoid arthritis 48).[28] Variation in genes associated with autoimmune diseases may improve PPV in combination with specific associated HLA alleles.

The mechanistic roles of the viruses in the initiation or perpetuation of T-cell mediated ADRs are complex and have been proposed to involve stimulation of virus-specific T cells. HHV-4 Epstein–Barr virus (EBV) (for ampicillin),[29] HHV-5 cytomegalovirus (CMV) (for sulfonamides and aminopenicillins),[30] HHV-6 herpes lymphotropic virus (for carbamazepine),[31] and human immunodeficiency virus (HIV) (for sulfamethoxazole/trimethoprim or sulfadiazine/pyrimethamine)[32] have been shown to be associated with drug hypersensitivity. It should be noted that there is no link between abacavir hypersensitivity and HIV infection because abacavir is not typically administered to uninfected individuals. Risk values such as PPV may be improved by consideration of the necessary HLA allele (strongly associated with drug hypersensitivity) combined with activation of one or several of these viruses.

POSITIVE PREDICTIVE VALUE MAY BE IMPROVED BASED ON A PHARMACOGENETIC TEST OF MULTIPLE GENE VARIANTS ASSOCIATED WITH RISK

Because multiple HLA alleles have been associated with hypersensitivities to the same drug (**Table 2**), the authors asked if HLA alleles other than the most strongly associated (necessary) allele were associated with dapsone hypersensitivity syndrome. They compared HLA alleles of dapsone hypersensitivity patients with dapsone-tolerant patients expressing HLA-B*13:01. HLA typing by DNA sequencing was conducted for second field resolution for HLA-A, HLA-B, HLA-C, HLA-DRB1, HLA-DQA1, and HLADQB1 (all patients in the analysis expressed HLA-B*13:01). There were several independent HLA associations, including HLA-A*02:01, which was observed less frequently in dapsone hypersensitivity patients compared with HLA-B*13:01⁺ dapsone-tolerant control patients (see **Table 2**). These data suggest that HLA-A*02:01 had a protective effect on dapsone hypersensitivity syndrome in a Han Chinese population. HLA-A*02:01 may confer protection by several possible mechanisms. Presentation of pathogen epitopes by HLA-A*02:01 (eg, derived from virus antigens in infected cells such as EBV or CMV) may reduce drug hypersensitivity risk by eliciting T cells that protect from infection. Alternatively, tolerance mechanisms conferred by HLA-A*02:01 may protect individuals from drug hypersensitivity by negatively selecting dapsone-specific T cells. By combining HLA-B*13:01⁺ and HLA-A*02:01⁻ into a biomarker with clinical research calculators,[33] PPV (true positives/true positives + false positives) increased from 30.5% to 39.8% in ethnic Chinese (predominantly Han).[10] The 7.8% PPV reported[10] were calculated based on 1.4% prevalence of dapsone hypersensitivity syndrome. These data demonstrate that it is feasible to identify new markers that improve PPV and yield insight into possible mechanistic interactions that regulate drug hypersensitivity.

Table 2
HLA-A*02:01 was associated with protection from dapsone hypersensitivity syndrome in HLA-B*13:01 positive patients

	Case	Control	Sum
HLA-B*13:01+	65	148	213
HLA-B*13:01-	11	886	897
Sum	76	1034	1110
HLA-B*13:01+ HLA-A*02:01−	96	145	241
HLA-B*13:01+ HLA-A*02:01+	7	36	43
Sum	103	181	284

Parameter	Calculation	B*13:01+	B*13:01+ A*02:01-
P-value	Fisher exact test (two-tailed)	<0.0001	<0.0001
Odds ratio	$\dfrac{\text{true positives} \times \text{true negatives}}{\text{false positives} \times \text{false negatives}}$	35.3 (18.2–68.6)	3.4 (1.5–8.0)
Sensitivity (case accuracy)	$\dfrac{\text{true positives}}{\text{true positives} + \text{false negatives}}$	85.6%	93.2%
Specificity (control accuracy)	$\dfrac{\text{true negatives}}{\text{true negatives} + \text{false positives}}$	85.7%	29.9%
Balanced accuracy	$\dfrac{\text{sensitivity} + \text{specificity}}{2}$	85.7%	61.6%
PPV	$\dfrac{\text{true positives}}{\text{true positives} + \text{false positives}}$	30.5%	39.8%
NPV	$\dfrac{\text{true negatives}}{\text{true negatives} + \text{false negatives}}$	98.8%	83.7%

Data from Stricker D. BrightStat.com: free statistics online. Comput Methods Programs Biomed 2008;92(1):135–43.

THE FUTURE OF DRUG HYPERSENSITIVITY PREVENTION

Associations between individual HLA alleles with hypersensitivities to specific drugs permit development of pharmacogenetic tests that accurately define patients at high levels of risk (eg, HLA-B*57:01 for abacavir hypersensitivity syndrome). Pharmacogenetic tests based on single HLA alleles lack specificity because all patients expressing the drug-associated allele do not develop hypersensitivity reactions (PPV 3%–55%, see **Table 1**).[19] Pharmacogenetic tests based on single HLA alleles combined with additional biomarkers associated with drug hypersensitivity are expected to be more specific in defining patients at the highest levels of risk. Tests to predict risk that combine variants of genes involved in T cell/NK cell recognition, drug metabolism, and autoimmunity with multiple HLA alleles will likely be developed for use in multiple forms. Prognostic tests may use data derived from a combination method including whole genome genotyping, sequence-based HLA typing, and measurement of T-cell responsiveness ex vivo. As technology for whole genome analysis becomes increasingly economical, more data on genetic variants, including HLA types,[34,35] are expected to be linked to electronic medical records in a manner that warns physicians that their patients may be at high levels of risk for developing hypersensitivity reactions to specific drugs.

REFERENCES

1. Rive CM, Bourke J, Phillips EJ. Testing for drug hypersensitivity syndromes. Clin Biochem Rev 2013;34(1):15–38.
2. Bharadwaj M, Illing P, Theodossis A, et al. Drug hypersensitivity and human leukocyte antigens of the major histocompatibility complex. Annu Rev Pharmacol Toxicol 2011. https://doi.org/10.1146/annurev-pharmtox-010611-134701.
3. White KD, Chung WH, Hung SI, et al. Evolving models of the immunopathogenesis of T cell-mediated drug allergy: the role of host, pathogens, and drug response. J Allergy Clin Immunol 2015;136(2):219–34 [quiz: 235].
4. Pavlos R, Mallal S, Ostrov D, et al. T cell-mediated hypersensitivity reactions to drugs. Annu Rev Med 2015;66:439–54.
5. Mallal S, Nolan D, Witt C, et al. Association between presence of HLA-B*5701, HLA-DR7, and HLA-DQ3 and hypersensitivity to HIV-1 reverse-transcriptase inhibitor abacavir. Lancet 2002;359(9308):727–32.
6. Hetherington S, Hughes AR, Mosteller M, et al. Genetic variations in HLA-B region and hypersensitivity reactions to abacavir. Lancet 2002;359(9312):1121–2.
7. Chung WH, Hung SI, Hong HS, et al. Medical genetics: a marker for stevens-johnson syndrome. Nature 2004;428(6982):486.
8. Man CB, Kwan P, Baum L, et al. Association between HLA-B*1502 allele and anti-epileptic drug-induced cutaneous reactions in han Chinese. Epilepsia 2007; 48(5):1015–8.
9. Hung SI, Chung WH, Liou LB, et al. HLA-B*5801 allele as a genetic marker for severe cutaneous adverse reactions caused by allopurinol. Proc Natl Acad Sci U S A 2005;102(11):4134–9.
10. Zhang FR, Liu H, Irwanto A, et al. HLA-B*13:01 and the dapsone hypersensitivity syndrome. N Engl J Med 2013;369(17):1620–8.
11. Faulkner L, Meng X, Park BK, et al. The importance of hapten-protein complex formation in the development of drug allergy. Curr Opin Allergy Clin Immunol 2014;14(4):293–300.
12. Pichler WJ. The p-i concept: pharmacological interaction of drugs with immune receptors. World Allergy Organ J 2008;1(6):96–102.
13. Illing PT, Vivian JP, Dudek NL, et al. Immune self-reactivity triggered by drug-modified HLA-peptide repertoire. Nature 2012;486(7404):554–8.
14. Norcross MA, Luo S, Lu L, et al. Abacavir induces loading of novel self-peptides into HLA-B*57: 01: an autoimmune model for HLA-associated drug hypersensitivity. AIDS 2012. https://doi.org/10.1097/QAD.0b013e328355fe8f.
15. Ostrov DA, Grant BJ, Pompeu YA, et al. Drug hypersensitivity caused by alteration of the MHC-presented self-peptide repertoire. Proc Natl Acad Sci U S A 2012. https://doi.org/10.1073/pnas.1207934109.
16. Yerly D, Pompeu YA, Schutte RJ, et al. Structural elements recognized by abacavir-induced T cells. Int J Mol Sci 2017;18(7) [pii:E1464].
17. Mallal S, Phillips E, Carosi G, et al. HLA-B*5701 screening for hypersensitivity to abacavir. N Engl J Med 2008;358(6):568–79.
18. Phillips EJ, Chung WH, Mockenhaupt M, et al. Drug hypersensitivity: pharmacogenetics and clinical syndromes. J Allergy Clin Immunol 2011;127(3 Suppl): S60–6.
19. White KD, Abe R, Ardern-Jones M, et al. SJS/TEN 2017: building multidisciplinary networks to drive science and translation. J Allergy Clin Immunol Pract 2018;6(1): 38–69.

20. Denisov IG, Grinkova YV, Baylon JL, et al. Mechanism of drug-drug interactions mediated by human cytochrome P450 CYP3A4 monomer. Biochemistry 2015. https://doi.org/10.1021/acs.biochem.5b00079.
21. Ota T, Kamada Y, Hayashida M, et al. Combination analysis in genetic polymorphisms of drug-metabolizing enzymes CYP1A2, CYP2C9, CYP2C19, CYP2D6 and CYP3A5 in the Japanese population. Int J Med Sci 2015;12(1):78–82.
22. Ogese MO, Jenkins RE, Maggs JL, et al. Characterization of peroxidases expressed in human antigen presenting cells and analysis of the covalent binding of nitroso sulfamethoxazole to myeloperoxidase. Chem Res Toxicol 2015. https://doi.org/10.1021/tx500458k.
23. Lu SC. Glutathione synthesis. Biochim Biophys Acta 2013;1830(5):3143–53.
24. Tang W, Jiang YF, Ponnusamy M, et al. Role of Nrf2 in chronic liver disease. World J Gastroenterol 2014;20(36):13079–87.
25. Oetjens MT, Denny JC, Ritchie MD, et al. Assessment of a pharmacogenomic marker panel in a polypharmacy population identified from electronic medical records. Pharmacogenomics 2013;14(7):735–44.
26. Selvaraj S, Schmitt AD, Dixon JR, et al. Complete haplotype phasing of the MHC and KIR loci with targeted HaploSeq. BMC Genomics 2015;16:900.
27. Rajagopalan S, Long EO. Understanding how combinations of HLA and KIR genes influence disease. J Exp Med 2005;201(7):1025–9.
28. Parkes M, Cortes A, van Heel DA, et al. Genetic insights into common pathways and complex relationships among immune-mediated diseases. Nat Rev Genet 2013;14(9):661–73.
29. Shiohara T, Kano Y. A complex interaction between drug allergy and viral infection. Clin Rev Allergy Immunol 2007;33(1–2):124–33.
30. Smith KJ, Skelton HG, Yeager J, et al. Increased drug reactions in HIV-1-positive patients: a possible explanation based on patterns of immune dysregulation seen in HIV-1 disease. the military medical consortium for the advancement of retroviral research (MMCARR). Clin Exp Dermatol 1997;22(3):118–23.
31. Aihara Y, Ito SI, Kobayashi Y, et al. Carbamazepine-induced hypersensitivity syndrome associated with transient hypogammaglobulinaemia and reactivation of human herpesvirus 6 infection demonstrated by real-time quantitative polymerase chain reaction. Br J Dermatol 2003;149(1):165–9.
32. Eliaszewicz M, Flahault A, Roujeau JC, et al. Prospective evaluation of risk factors of cutaneous drug reactions to sulfonamides in patients with AIDS. J Am Acad Dermatol 2002;47(1):40–6.
33. Stricker D. BrightStat.com: free statistics online. Comput Methods Programs Biomed 2008;92(1):135–43.
34. Dalbeth N, Stamp LK, Merriman TR. The genetics of gout: towards personalised medicine? BMC Med 2017;15(1):108.
35. Ashley EA, Butte AJ, Wheeler MT, et al. Clinical assessment incorporating a personal genome. Lancet 2010;375(9725):1525–35.

Human Leukocyte Antigen and Disease Associations

A Broader Perspective

Mengkai Shieh, MD[a], Nilesh Chitnis, PhD[a], Dimitri Monos, PhD[b],*

KEYWORDS

- HLA • Next-generation sequencing • NGS • miRNA • Disease associations • MHC
- Complexity theory

KEY POINTS

- Genome-wide association studies have demonstrated the special significance of the major histocompatibility complex (MHC) region in disease susceptibility; this genomic region is associated with the highest number of diseases/single-nucleotide polymorphisms as compared with any other genomic region of comparable size.
- HLA molecules interact extensively with other genomic regions to carry out their functions, such as through microRNAs and epistatic interactions.
- The advent of high-throughput sequencing technologies provides a new opportunity for developing insights into the association of the many HLA alleles with numerous diseases.
- The reported associations of HLA alleles with diseases may involve not only the antigen recognition domains of the binding site but also other protein elements like transmembrane and cytoplasmic regions or genomic sequences of intronic segments that code for microRNAs and control the expression of multiple cellular pathways.
- Detailed and accurate sequencing of the MHC in a haplotypic form will be necessary to elucidate the interactive relationships of the MHC genes among themselves or with other genomic regions that generate a disease phenotype.

INTRODUCTION

Many diseases, with a phenotype suggesting the involvement of the immune response, are frequently found to have an association with specific HLA alleles. Identifying the exact molecular mechanisms by which the HLA molecules are involved in the pathophysiology of these diseases remains challenging. Significant progress has been

Disclosure Statement: The authors have nothing to disclose.
[a] Department of Pathology and Laboratory Medicine, The Children's Hospital of Philadelphia, Abramson Research Center, Room 707, 3615 Civic Center Boulevard, Philadelphia, PA 19104, USA; [b] Department of Pathology and Laboratory Medicine, The Children's Hospital of Philadelphia, Perelman School of Medicine, University of Pennsylvania, Abramson Research Center, Room 707A, 3615 Civic Center Boulevard, Philadelphia, PA 19104, USA
* Corresponding author.
E-mail address: monosd@email.chop.edu

Clin Lab Med 38 (2018) 679–693
https://doi.org/10.1016/j.cll.2018.07.001
0272-2712/18/© 2018 Elsevier Inc. All rights reserved.

labmed.theclinics.com

made toward elucidating the molecular complexes formed by specific HLA alleles and peptides that trigger an undesirable immune response, such as in celiac disease or adverse reactions to medications like abacavir, but the exact HLA-peptide complexes that trigger an immune response for many HLA-associated diseases remain unknown.

The traditional approach for establishing the association of specific diseases with HLA alleles/structures has been to assess the differential presence of HLA alleles in a disease versus a control population, thereby establishing correlation of particular HLA elements with susceptibility or protection. This approach has provided valuable information regarding the role of specific HLA alleles/structures, but invariably, it has been found that the complete story is always more complicated; the HLA molecules appear to be necessary components of a process, but they alone are insufficient to wholly explain the observed phenomena. Meanwhile, in the last decade or so, through a different approach that is hypothesis agnostic, in which no specific hypothesis is proposed regarding the mechanism of a disease, multiple regions throughout the genome are reported to be associated with different diseases. The genomic regions identified are designated by specific single-nucleotide polymorphisms (SNPs), and the studies are called genome-wide association studies (GWAS). The evidence from such studies thus far has indicated that the broader HLA region, named the major histocompatibility complex (MHC), is associated by far with the largest number of diseases in the human genome, compared with any other region of equivalent size (4 Mbp) (**Fig. 1**). Therefore, the MHC has been recognized as the most important region of

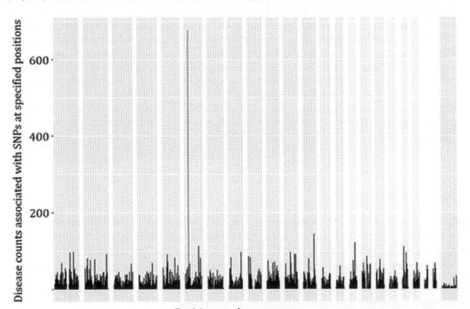

Fig. 1. Density of diseases associated with specific SNPs in the human genome (4-Mbp bins). Disease counts associated with SNPs located in the MHC are colored red. The MHC (chr6: 29–33 Mb = 4 Mb) includes ~260 genes, about half of which are involved in the immune response, 884 unique loci associated with 479 unique traits/diseases, and 112 unique disease phenotypes. (*Data from* MacArthur J, Bowler E, Cerezo M, et al. The new NHGRI-EBI catalog of published genome-wide association studies (GWAS Catalog). Nucleic Acids Res 2017;45(D1):D896–901; and Clark PM, Kunkel M, Monos DS. The dichotomy between disease phenotype databases and the implications for understanding complex diseases involving the major histocompatibility complex. Int J Immunogenet 2015;42(6):413–22.)

the human genome in relation to disease susceptibility.[1] It is noteworthy that the region seems to be associated not only with diseases of an immune-related etiology but also with diseases that have no apparent connection with the immune response. In addition, diseases associated with specific HLA alleles appear to be associated with multiple SNPs both within and outside of the MHC, suggesting interplay of several, if not numerous, genomic regions in the manifestations of such diseases. It is noteworthy that these regions very frequently represent noncoding regions[2] and very infrequently represent exonic regions. Therefore, the emerging picture is one of high complexity in which the MHC is associated with many diseases that may or may not involve the HLA genes. Furthermore, even if and when the HLA genes are involved, there exist other genomic regions outside of the MHC that contribute to the disease phenotype. Delineating the interactive relationships of these genomic regions requires a reliable and efficient sequencing methodology that would provide detailed genomic characterization of these regions (HLA genes, MHC region, and others), including all coding and noncoding sequences, followed by a sophisticated bioinformatics approach that ensures proper analysis of a rather voluminous set of data. The purpose of this article is to introduce a new approach to analyzing the association of HLAs with diseases in which the HLA genes are treated as an integral, although not sole, component of a highly complex interaction that involves the broader MHC region as well as other genomic regions, which collectively establish the disease phenotype.

THE IMPACT OF TECHNOLOGY

HLA genes are the most polymorphic set of genes found in humans, estimated to contain on the order of millions of alleles per locus.[3] Besides the extreme HLA allelic variation, the broader genomic context of the HLAs, namely the MHC, is itself characterized by high complexity, with numerous SNPs and genes in extensive linkage disequilibrium as well as many structural variations of all kinds (eg, inversions, deletions, and duplications). The high gene density of the region only adds to its complexity, and about half of the region consists of repeats. In the past, this region resisted detailed characterization, and only through intense efforts of cloning and Sanger sequencing could one gain a glimpse at its complexity through the sequencing of several homozygous B lymphoblastoid cell lines (BLCLs). The MHC region of two of these BLCLs (PGF and COX) has been fully sequenced[4] and constitutes reference sequences for the human reference genome.[5] With the advent of high-throughput/next-generation sequencing (NGS), significant progress has been made in the characterization of the HLA genes,[6–10] with several vendors now offering commercial solutions for HLA typing. One now can attain complete characterization of the HLA genes, including both exonic and intronic regions, using relatively simplified protocols and at a reasonable cost. However, the progress made on the thorough and accurate characterization of the entire MHC, a segment of approximately 4-M bases, has been rather incremental and slow. Efforts to characterize the MHC from whole genome sequencing data (using Illumina short-read technology) have generally proven to be ineffective, because they have usually relied on reference-based assembly, which is problematic for such a highly polymorphic region as the MHC, resulting in gaps, discontinuities, and inaccurate sequences. The most recent advances have included approaches that involve whole genome sequencing using short-read technologies of either family trios[11] or a combination of both long-read and short-read technologies of individual subjects.[12] The common denominator for both approaches is the requirement of whole genome sequencing before the MHC haplotypes are generated, rendering these approaches impractical and cost inefficient for studying many subjects.

To address this cost and efficiency challenge, methods that selectively target and sequence the 4 Mb of the MHC have recently been developed.[13,14] The approach by Norman and colleagues[13] involves only homozygous DNA samples, and as a result, it is not generally applicable to the generation of haplotypes from heterozygous samples. The authors' laboratory has developed an approach that includes selective targeting of the MHC, capturing long DNA fragments of 10 to 20 Kb, and subsequent sequencing on PacBio. The resulting sequenced fragments range from a few Kb to more than 20 Kb, with an average of about 5 Kb. The size of the fragments allow for a de novo–based assembly process generating very accurate assembly (99.9%) and significant coverage (98.2%) (Timothy M, Taishan HU, Dimitri M, unpublished data, 2018). Further progress in this particular domain will allow for efficient sequencing of the MHC in order to investigate various disease categories. Such complete sequencing information will then form the basis for exhaustive and comprehensive comparisons, enabling the identification and analysis of detailed genomic features of relevance, which have hitherto been opaque to precise and detailed inquiry. The need for such detailed and thorough sequencing is underscored by a report[2] on GWAS data, which indicates that 90% of causal variants of autoimmune diseases are located in noncoding regions. These types of findings emphasize the need for thorough, detailed, and accurate sequencing of the MHC, as well as other SNP-containing genomic regions associated with diseases of interest.

THE POTENTIAL ROLE OF microRNAs

In order to explore the functional significance of noncoding regions within the MHC, the presence of functional microRNAs (miRNAs) encoded within the noncoding regions of the MHC was sought. Among the 12 miRNA precursors reported to be present within the MHC, one (miR-6891) was located within intron 4 of HLA-B. Upon investigating the biological role of miR-6891 by in vitro inhibition of the expression of miR-6891-5p by anti–miR-6891-5p, it was found that this particular miRNA controls more than 200 transcripts in COX BLCLs, affecting a large number of metabolic pathways, including various immune response networks.[15] One of the targeted transcripts was the immunoglobulin A (IgA) heavy chain. The authors validated that miR-6891-5p mediates posttranscriptional regulation of immunoglobulin heavy chain transcripts and showed that in BLCLs from IgA-immunodeficient patients that express neither IgA messenger RNA (mRNA) nor protein, upon modulating (reducing) the expression levels of miR-6891-5p, the expression levels of both the IgA transcript and its respective protein were restored.[15] These findings demonstrate that "noncoding" sequences of HLA genes may contain regulatory potential, with the ability to influence immunologic processes, and thereby become elements of association with diseases. To evaluate further the presence of additional miRNAs within the MHC, the authors studied 2 BLCLs with known MHC sequences (PGF and COX) and identified, using deep RNA sequencing, the miRNAs encoded by the two cell lines. The authors' analysis identified 89 novel miRNA transcripts, 48 of which undergo Dicer-dependent biogenesis and are loaded onto the Argonaute silencing complex. Several of the identified mature miRNA and pre-miRNA transcripts are unique to specific MHC haplotypes and overlap common SNPs.[16] Furthermore, 43 of the 89 identified novel miRNA transcripts lie within linkage disequilibrium blocks that contain a disease-associated SNP. These disease-associated SNPs are associated with 65 unique disease phenotypes, suggesting that these transcripts may play a role in the etiology of numerous diseases associated with the MHC. Additional in silico analysis reveals the potential for up to thousands of pre-miRNA–encoding loci to be present within the MHC, where encoded miRNAs may be differentially expressed in different cell types and at different developmental stages.[16] Considering that each miRNA can control multiple transcripts affecting multiple metabolic pathways and that the MHC potentially encodes a very large number of miRNAs, the potential impact of these MHC-derived miRNAs in disease susceptibility appears quite significant.

The above examples represent cases in which miRNAs encoded by the MHC may exhibit a significant functional impact and therefore may influence a particular disease phenotype. The literature, furthermore, contains many examples of miRNAs encoded by other parts of the genome that interact with sequences of the MHC, also with important implications for many physiologic and also pathologic phenotypes.

One such example is miR-148a (chromosome 7), which influences the expression of HLA-C, depending on polymorphisms in the 3′ untranslated region (UTR). Binding of miR-148a to its target site results in lower surface expression of HLA-C relative to those alleles that escape its binding. Interestingly, the high expression levels of some HLA-C alleles and associated lack of binding of miR-148a to those 3′ UTR variants associates strongly with better human immunodeficiency virus control and greater risk of Crohn's disease.[17–19]

MiR-148a is also involved, together with miR-152 (chromosome 17), in regulating HLA-G expression by binding to the 3′ UTR of its transcript.[20] HLA-G is a nonclassical HLA class-Ib molecule expressed mainly in the extravillous cytotrophoblasts (EVT) of the placenta. The expression of HLA-G on these fetal cells protects the EVT cells from immune rejection and is therefore important for a healthy pregnancy. It has been shown that in the placenta both miR-148a and miR-152 miRNAs are expressed at relatively low levels, compared with other healthy tissues, which likely contributes to the high levels of HLA-G mRNA in the placenta.[20] Other studies show that miR-365 also targets HLA-G at its 3′ UTR, thus repressing its expression.[21] The expression of miR-365 may play an important role in human placental development and in immunoprotection of the semiallogenic embryo by coordinating, in concert with other miRNAs, the proper levels of HLA-G expression in the trophoblast. Furthermore, HLA-G regulation by miRNA-133a (miR-133a-1, miR-133a-2, and miR-133b found on chromosomes 18, 20, and 6, respectively) is implicated in the pathogenesis of recurrent pregnancy loss.[22]

Alterations in HLA-G expression may be implicated in other disease processes as well. MiR-148– and miR-152–mediated regulation of HLA-G has been proposed as a risk factor in asthma,[23] and the modulation of HLA-G expression by miR-148a, miR-152, miR-548, miR-628-5p, and miR-133a has been shown to influence tumor progression.[24–30] This modulation of HLA-G expression levels has been closely associated with various tumor escape pathways and mechanisms.

Another example of a miRNA that influences the immune response is miR-9 (chromosome 1). This miRNA has been shown to modulate the expression of interferon (IFN)-induced genes and MHC class I molecules (HLA-B, HLA-C, HLA-F, and HLA-H) in nasopharyngeal carcinoma (NPC), suggesting a novel role of miR-9 in linking inflammation with cancer.[31] The exact role of miR-9 dysregulation in the pathogenesis of NPC is unclear, but its influence on class I molecules is most likely achieved through interaction with the 3′ UTR regions of these genes and therefore constitutes a further example of the significant role that miRNAs play in regulating HLA genes and influencing disease development and host response.

The data presented above demonstrate some of the unique and important features of miRNAs as they interact with their targets within the MHC, regulate HLA gene expression, and affect various phenotypes. The emerging picture is one in which distinct sequences found across the human genome—in the above examples, these represent miRNA sequences—appear to influence gene expression and regulation of HLAs, as well as of other distant genes. The involvement of non-HLA sequences in HLA-mediated diseases does not negate the important role of the HLA genes themselves in disease pathophysiology. HLA molecules, as antigen presenting molecules, may be seen as critical and necessary building blocks, but their functionality or effects may be significantly altered by various intra- and extra-MHC genomic sequences (eg, in the form of miRNAs and perhaps other RNA species or molecules). The emerging picture of a potentially significant role of dynamic and varied HLA expression, regulated by direct RNA products of near and distant genomic sequences, adds yet another intriguing layer of complexity to this already highly polymorphic MHC region and highlights the rich complexity of genomic interactions in human health and disease.

EXAMPLES OF EPISTATIC INTERACTIONS INVOLVING THE MAJOR HISTOCOMPATIBILITY COMPLEX

There are many examples in which diseases associated with SNPs within the MHC have additional associations with SNPs located outside of the MHC, with such associations being dictated by epistatic interactions. In these cases, the combined presence of the associated SNPs confers a higher overall risk for the disease. Examples of gene-gene epistatic interactions among susceptibility loci involving the MHC have been reported in systemic lupus erythematosus (MHC with CTLA4 and IRF5),[32] Bechet disease (HLA-B*51 and endoplasmic reticulum aminopeptidase-1 [ERAP1]),[33] ankylosing spondylitis (HLAs and ERAP1),[34] Sjogren syndrome (HLA DR3 and RCA alpha block-complement regulatory genes or proinflammatory receptor P2X7),[35,36] inflammatory bowel disease (HLA-C and ERAP1),[37] Chagas disease (MHC and IL-10),[38] psoriasis (MHC and IL12B, LCE),[39] and others. The exact mechanisms and interactions that produce the disease phenotypes remain largely unknown. As the independent contributions of the involved genomic regions are better appreciated and the complex pathways by which these regions may interact are elucidated, it is expected that a deeper insight will be developed to explain the heightened, combined risk of these SNP-associated regions.

HUMAN LEUKOCYTE ANTIGEN GENOTYPING BY NEXT-GENERATION SEQUENCING

Technological advances in DNA sequencing have provided a unique opportunity for significantly enhancing the understanding of the possible role of HLAs in diseases. Unquestionably, NGS has enabled the complete characterization of the HLA genes, enabling the assessment of regions not traditionally characterized by legacy methods, such as intronic regions, additional exonic regions, as well as 5′ and 3′ UTRs. Data have accumulated suggesting that all of these regions, far beyond simply the regions corresponding to antigen recognition domains, play an important physiologic role and therefore are likely to be relevant in the association of certain alleles with diseases and other traits (see later discussion regarding the information content and interactions of all genomic regions as revealed by complexity theory). Our scientific community is at a stage of exploring these regions at an ever-increasing depth in order to discover their biological relevance and functionality. The authors examined earlier the significant role of 3′ UTR sequences in the context of miRNA interactions and effects. Recent literature also documents the significant role of the sequences encoding the transmembrane and cytoplasmic regions of HLA class II genes.[40–43] Intronic sequences are also relevant because they harbor sequences that may affect alternative splicing and may encode such sequences as the mirtron miRNA-6891-5p, found in intron 4 of HLA-B, which appears to influence the expression of more than 200 transcripts in the cell and may thus influence numerous types of pathways, including critical immunologic processes, as previously mentioned.[15] It is very likely that additional intronic sequences from the HLA genes will prove to have significant roles. However, besides the advantage afforded by using NGS for the characterization of the HLA genes, NGS, as a technology that allows for the high-throughput sequencing of genomic sequences, creates another advantage that is not always readily appreciated. This advantage is the high depth of sequencing coverage attainable by NGS, which translates to a reliable detection of minor genomic events. This property of NGS technology became quite apparent in the following study of acquired aplastic anemia (aAA).

aAA is an acquired bone marrow failure syndrome caused by autoimmune destruction of early hematopoietic cells and is associated with myelodysplastic syndrome and leukemia. Although its exact pathogenesis is unknown, aAA is thought to be driven by HLA-restricted T-cell immunity. Using a combination of targeted deep sequencing of HLA class I genes and SNP array genotyping, the authors screened 66 patients with aAA for somatic HLA class I allele loss. They found somatic HLA loss in 11 patients (17%), with 13 loss-of-function mutations in HLA-A*33:03, HLA-A*68:01, HLA-B*14:02, and HLA-B*40:02 alleles. Three patients had more than one mutation on a single HLA allele. Mutations were detected at a frequency of 1.6% to 20.1%, with 1% being the commonly accepted level of nonspecific noise. Software adjustments and a depth of close to 5,000 to 10,000 reads is necessary for a detected mutation to be deemed credible. Presumably, clones aborting certain HLA alleles gain a survival advantage and perpetuate themselves as clones that increase gradually in numbers. The finding of recurrent HLA class I mutations provides compelling evidence for a predominant HLA class I–driven autoimmunity in aAA and establishes a novel link between immunogenetics and clonal evolution of patients with aAA.[44] The ability to gain powerful insights into such disease processes as aAA by application of NGS technology has clearly demonstrated an important aspect of the impact that NGS technology has brought upon the field. It has allowed the detection of rare mutational events that were previously unattainable with legacy methods. These findings pave the way for identifying the specific HLA molecules involved in disease processes as well as eventually the associated antigens involved in the autoimmune response.

THE ROLE OF HUMAN LEUKOCYTE ANTIGENS IN CANCER AND CANCER IMMUNOTHERAPIES

The authors have chosen to present two aspects of the way in which HLAs are implicated in cancer-related processes. One relates to the role of HLAs in cancer pathogenesis, and the other is the role of HLAs in cancer immunotherapies.

Immune evasion is a hallmark of cancer. The HLA molecules are central to immune surveillance, and thus, losing the ability to present neoantigens through HLAs can facilitate immune evasion. HLA expression is known to be suppressed in many cancers. Changes in HLA expression come about either through a direct effect on the regulatory machinery of HLA expression or via disturbances in the antigen processing and presentation system. Perturbations via both mechanistic pathways can influence the expression of intact and functional HLAs on the cell surface. Examples of downregulation of HLA class I expression have been observed in lung cancer where allele-specific loss (loss of heterozygosity)[45] or significant reduction in expression of certain alleles is observed.[46] Another mechanism of transcriptional inactivation reported to influence HLA class I expression at both the protein and the mRNA levels in esophageal squamous cell carcinoma is through hypermethylation of the promoter regions of the HLA class I genes.[47] In addition, activation of the mitogen-activated protein kinase pathway has also been shown to suppress components of the MHC class I and antigen presentation machinery and thus promote tumor development in multiple cancers.[48] Malignant cells may also have multiple HLA class I antigen–processing machinery defects. These defects include loss of tapasin or selective silencing of HLA-A3 gene responsiveness to INF-γ.[49] Associations have also been reported between the antigen processing machinery and cervical carcinoma. One study found partial HLA class I loss to be significantly associated with decreased 5-year overall survival and decreased 5-year disease-free survival. They also found that downregulation of components of the antigen processing machinery was significantly associated with HLA class I downregulation.[50] In another study involving primary and metastatic lesions of head and neck squamous cell carcinoma, it was found that expression levels of Transporter associated with Antigen Processing molecules, TAP1 and TAP2, together with tapasin, were coordinately downregulated with HLA class I antigen in both primary and metastatic lesions, with significantly lower levels found in metastatic lesions as compared with autologous primary lesions.[51] The downregulation of HLA class I antigen in metastatic lesions was also associated with reduced disease-free survival.

The limited number of studies and examples presented above already amply illustrate the multiplicity of metabolic points at which a perturbation can result in reduced cell surface expression of HLA class I molecules and thus allow cancerous cells to evade immune surveillance and remain undetectable by the immune response. Knowing the exact mechanisms of such types of reduced HLA class I expression would establish the foundations for developing therapeutic interventions that restore cell surface expression of HLA class I molecules.

HLA molecules, besides being implicated in mechanisms of immune surveillance evasion by cancer cells, are also involved in processes that influence immunotherapy approaches. Immunotherapy is a broad category of cancer therapies that use the body's immune system to fight cancer cells. One category includes cytokines, vaccines, and infusions of engineered T cells, whereas the other category includes the use of monoclonal antibodies to target and inhibit certain immune-suppressing proteins expressed by cancer cells. HLA molecules, based on recently published reports, appear to be somehow relevant to both categories of immunotherapy.

Development of vaccines requires knowledge of the antigenic entities that will form the stimulant for the immune response. These antigenic entities (peptides) form complexes with HLA class I molecules that stimulate CD8$^+$ T cells. It is widely accepted that the ligandome originating from cancer-associated antigens and bound to HLA molecules has the potential to become the basis for effective peptide vaccines for cancer immunotherapy. Many examples in the literature identify ligands originating from various cancers, such as prostate cancer,[52] acute myeloid leukemia,[53,54] glioblastoma,[55] lung cancer,[56,57] esophageal cancer,[57] chronic myeloid leukemia,[58] and ovarian cancer.[59,60]

The above-mentioned studies reveal antigenic peptides that are generated during the progression of a tumor, deducing that these peptides may form the basis for vaccine development. However, a recent study[61] raises the possibility that in actuality there may be an HLA-dependent immunoediting process of oncogenic mutations that occurs in tumor cells, resulting in antigenic peptides that are not presented as effectively by the HLAs to the immune system, allowing the escape of tumor cells expressing these antigenic peptides. The results suggest that the HLA-bound peptides from tumor cells may not necessarily be the best choice for developing a vaccine, at least for the specific individual with a given HLA genotype, and that understanding the relationships/links between HLAs and particular tumors is critical. It appears that HLA-based precision strategies will be necessary for cancer prevention and immunotherapy.

In addition, it appears that HLAs may also be involved in the second category of immunotherapy, which involves the usage of antibodies directed against certain immune checkpoint proteins that inhibit T-cell function and are overexpressed by some cancer cells. These therapeutic antibodies, jointly named immune checkpoint inhibitors, target programmed cell death protein 1, its ligand, or cytotoxic T lymphocyte–associated protein 4 and thereby increase the activity of CD8$^+$ T cells. The cancer cells inactivate this apoptotic pathway by overexpressing the inhibitory checkpoint proteins, allowing survival of the cancer cells, whereas the therapeutic antibodies inactivate these overexpressed inhibitory proteins, thereby allowing cytotoxic CD8$^+$ T cells to eliminate the target cancer cells. Patient outcome and response to the drugs (antibodies), however, are not consistent. It was recently reported that immune checkpoint inhibitors lead to improved survival in those with increased heterozygosity of HLA class I alleles.[62] The study also reported that melanoma patients with the HLA-B44 supertype had extended survival, whereas the HLA-B62 supertype (including HLA-B*15:01) and those with somatic loss of heterozygosity at HLA class I had poorer outcomes. Additionally, HLA-B*15:01 was found in the same study, using molecular dynamics simulations, to contain elements that may impair CD8$^+$ T-cell recognition of neoantigens. Such types of findings demonstrate the vital influence of HLAs in immunotherapeutic approaches and the need to elucidate their roles further for continued advancement of immunotherapy.

A MULTIDISCIPLINARY APPROACH INVOLVING COMPLEXITY THEORY FOR THE STUDY OF THE MAJOR HISTOCOMPATIBILITY COMPLEX

Upon the completion of the Human Genome Project, it was recognized that nearly 99% of the genome does not encode proteins. An intense search in the following decade through the ENCODE (ENCyclopedia Of DNA Elements) project revealed that a significant portion of the genome encodes for RNA transcripts, transcriptional regulator binding sites, and chromatin states in many cell types.[63] It is recognized that there are additional functional elements that are still unknown, likely playing important roles in the physiology of the cell. The ENCODE project continues to delineate the role and interactive relationships of the different genomic elements through experimental and computational approaches.[63] For example, researchers have developed computational methods to identify and characterize DNA motifs throughout the genome using methods borrowed from the fields of Pattern Recognition and Complexity Theory. In the last few decades, nonlinear dynamical analysis and nonextensive statistical mechanics–based methods[64–67] have become semantic tools in the analysis of raw data of various complex systems. These tools from the science of nonlinear complex systems can be used to describe the basic dynamic characteristics of a complex system such as the human genome and may be used to understand the very structure and organization of the human genome. The authors have recently used approaches from complexity theory to interrogate the coding and noncoding regions of the MHC, in search of information content and interactive relationships that may exist among the exonic, intronic, and intergenic regions.[68] The authors demonstrated that MHC sequences, whether exonic, intronic, or intergenic, include varying levels and patterns of information encoding and contain specific relationships of genes with intergenic regions in which the lower the number of genes in a region, the less the complexity and information content of the intergenic region. The authors showed the significance of intergenic regions by providing quantitative measures of information content and complexity patterns as well as by correlating aspects of their information encoding dynamics with those of the other genomic regions. The results most likely are relevant to the whole genome and not only to the MHC. Meanwhile, GWAS studies indicate that most trait-associated loci, including ones contributing to diseases and susceptibility, lie outside of protein-coding regions.[2] The important role that noncoding regions play and the way in which they interact with other regions suggest that noncoding disease-associated variants of the MHC may arise as a result of their connection to functional elements, such as miRNAs. However, they may also indicate connection to functional elements of an as yet unknown or less understood nature, which is an area that requires further investigation. The authors hope that their novel analytical approach, which uses concepts from complexity theory and computational sciences, will be instructive and reveal patterns, information content, and relationships that exist among different genomic sequences, which in turn will help us to better comprehend the association of the MHC with diseases.

SUMMARY

Although the key role of the HLA molecules is antigen presentation, and although the antigen recognition domain and its corresponding gene sequence remain of undeniable significance in immunity, accumulated knowledge regarding the extended areas of the HLA molecules and further genomic regions of the HLA genes has enriched the understanding of the many ways in which the basic antigen recognition functionality and role can be shaped and altered to produce varying phenotypes. Whether a T-cell receptor or a killer cell immunoglobulin-like receptor is interacting with an HLA molecule, its overall effect and function can be influenced both spatially and temporally by the alteration of HLA molecule expression and peptides bound. Expression can be affected by MHC or non-MHC genomic sequences (eg, in the form of miRNAs) that interact with response elements of HLA genes, affecting expression levels; peptides available for binding can be affected by the antigen presentation machinery of the cell. Other further changes in the transmembrane or cytoplasmic regions of the HLA molecules can affect activation of the engaged cells. The significance of HLA genes in cancer and cancer immunotherapies is being increasingly realized, and there exists an unequivocal notion that HLAs will play a major role as we move forward with individualized approaches to cancer prevention and immunotherapy. GWAS studies have underlined the significance of the MHC region in a wide range of diseases and remind us that HLA molecules do not operate in a vacuum but rather interact extensively with other genomic regions to carry out their functions. Considering that the MHC region is the only 4-Mb region of the genome associated with such a large number of traits and diseases, it is possible that the MHC includes genomic elements and genes with functionalities of which we are yet unaware. The advent of high-throughput sequencing technologies, allowing the massive, thorough, and accurate characterization of the HLA genes—and soon the entire 4-Mb MHC region—has enabled our community to ask more questions regarding the genomic organization of the HLA genes, as well as that of the numerous other genes encoded by the MHC. These technologies have unquestionably provided opportunities and insights previously unattainable. Because of such advances and new possibilities, our field has been undergoing a profound paradigm shift. In the past, our community searched for causal relationships between elements within the MHC and immunologic conditions, intuitively based on the presence of HLA genes in the region. Now we may almost turn the whole approach on its head and say: if there is *any* disease that is found to be associated with an SNP within the MHC, we have reason to search for a possible immunologic basis of that disease, regardless of the apparent phenotype and any perceived nonrelationship of that disease with the immune response. Examples of diseases associated with MHC SNPs that do not have obvious connections to the immune response include such neurologic diseases as Parkinson, Alzheimer, or even schizophrenia. Nevertheless, these diseases, it has been recently shown, include elements of the immune response that may contribute to disease susceptibility.[69–72] Finally, the approach the authors have recently taken in analyzing genomic sequences by applying methodologies and analysis approaches borrowed from the domain of complexity theory has provided entirely new insights into the encoding of information in different types of genomic regions, whether coding or noncoding, and has revealed specific quantifiable patterns by which the embedded information in these separate genomic regions is related. The remarkable agreement of this technique with findings from the ENCODE project, which has been ongoing for more than 10 years now, is inspiring and has demonstrated the noteworthy potential of such a novel approach in corroborating and shedding new light on the findings and results of such major projects as ENCODE.

REFERENCES

1. Clark PM, Kunkel M, Monos DS. The dichotomy between disease phenotype databases and the implications for understanding complex diseases involving the major histocompatibility complex. Int J Immunogenet 2015;42(6):413–22.
2. Farh KK-H, Marson A, Zhu J, et al. Genetic and epigenetic fine mapping of causal autoimmune disease variants. Nature 2015;518(7539):337–43.
3. Klitz W, Hedrick P, Louis EJ. New reservoirs of HLA alleles: pools of rare variants enhance immune defense. Trends Genet 2012;28(10):480–6.
4. Horton R, Gibson R, Coggill P, et al. Variation analysis and gene annotation of eight MHC haplotypes: the MHC haplotype project. Immunogenetics 2008;60(1):1–18.
5. UCL. MHC haplotype project. UCL cancer institute. 2017. Available at: https://www.ucl.ac.uk/cancer/research/department-cancer-biology/medical-genomics/medical-genomics-past-projects/mhc-haplotype. Accessed May 24, 2018.
6. Gabriel C, Danzer M, Hackl C, et al. Rapid high-throughput human leukocyte antigen typing by massively parallel pyrosequencing for high-resolution allele identification. Hum Immunol 2009;70(11):960–4.
7. Lind C, Ferriola D, Mackiewicz K, et al. Next-generation sequencing: the solution for high-resolution, unambiguous human leukocyte antigen typing. Hum Immunol 2010;71(10):1033–42.
8. Holcomb CL, Hoeglund B, Anderson MW, et al. A multi-site study using high-resolution HLA genotyping by next generation sequencing. Tissue Antigens 2011;77(3):206–17.
9. Duke JL, Lind C, Mackiewicz K, et al. Determining performance characteristics of an NGS-based HLA typing method for clinical applications: Determining performance characteristics for NGS-based HLA typing. HLA 2016;87(3):141–52.
10. Gandhi MJ, Ferriola D, Huang Y, et al. Targeted next-generation sequencing for human leukocyte antigen typing in a clinical laboratory: metrics of relevance and considerations for its successful implementation. Arch Pathol Lab Med 2017;141(6):806–12.
11. Maretty L, Jensen JM, Petersen B, et al. Sequencing and de novo assembly of 150 genomes from Denmark as a population reference. Nature 2017; 548(7665):87–91.

12. Jain M, Koren S, Miga KH, et al. Nanopore sequencing and assembly of a human genome with ultra-long reads. Nat Biotechnol 2018;36(4):338–45.
13. Norman PJ, Norberg SJ, Guethlein LA, et al. Sequences of 95 human *MHC* haplotypes reveal extreme coding variation in genes other than highly polymorphic *HLA class I* and II. Genome Res 2017;27(5):813–23.
14. Dapprich J, Ferriola D, Mackiewicz K, et al. The next generation of target capture technologies - large DNA fragment enrichment and sequencing determines regional genomic variation of high complexity. BMC Genomics 2016;17:486.
15. Chitnis N, Clark PM, Kamoun M, et al. An expanded role for HLA genes: HLA-B encodes a microRNA that regulates IgA and other immune response transcripts. Front Immunol 2017;8:583.
16. Clark PM, Chitnis N, Shieh M, et al. Novel and haplotype specific micrornas encoded by the major histocompatibility complex. Sci Rep 2018;8(1):3832.
17. Kulkarni S, Savan R, Qi Y, et al. Differential microRNA regulation of HLA-C expression and its association with HIV control. Nature 2011;472(7344):495–8.
18. Kulkarni S, Qi Y, O'hUigin C, et al. Genetic interplay between HLA-C and MIR148A in HIV control and Crohn disease. Proc Natl Acad Sci 2013;110(51):20705–10.
19. Naranbhai V, Carrington M. Host genetic variation and HIV disease: from mapping to mechanism. Immunogenetics 2017;69(8–9):489–98.
20. Manaster I, Goldman-Wohl D, Greenfield C, et al. MiRNA-mediated control of HLA-G expression and function. Bobé P, ed. PLoS One 2012;7(3):e33395.
21. Mori A, Nishi H, Sasaki T, et al. HLA-G expression is regulated by miR-365 in trophoblasts under hypoxic conditions. Placenta 2016;45:37–41.
22. Wang X, Li B, Wang J, et al. Evidence that miR-133a causes recurrent spontaneous abortion by reducing HLA-G expression. Reprod Biomed Online 2012;25(4):415–24.
23. Tan Z, Randall G, Fan J, et al. Allele-specific targeting of microRNAs to HLA-G and risk of asthma. Am J Hum Genet 2007;81(4):829–34.
24. Chen Q, Luo G, Zhang X. MiR-148a modulates HLA-G expression and influences tumor apoptosis in esophageal squamous cell carcinoma. Exp Ther Med 2017;14(5):4448–52.
25. Sun J, Chu H, Ji J, et al. Long non-coding RNA HOTAIR modulates HLA-G expression by absorbing miR-148a in human cervical cancer. Int J Oncol 2016;49(3):943–52.
26. Jasinski-Bergner S, Reches A, Stoehr C, et al. Identification of novel microRNAs regulating HLA-G expression and investigating their clinical relevance in renal cell carcinoma. Oncotarget 2016;7(18):26866–78.
27. Guan Z, Song B, Liu F, et al. TGF-β induces HLA-G expression through inhibiting miR-152 in gastric cancer cells. J Biomed Sci 2015;22(1):107.
28. Bian X, Si Y, Zhang M, et al. Down-expression of miR-152 lead to impaired antitumor effect of NK via upregulation of HLA-G. Tumor Biol 2016;37(3):3749–56.
29. Song B, Guan Z, Liu F, et al. Long non-coding RNA HOTAIR promotes HLA-G expression via inhibiting miR-152 in gastric cancer cells. Biochem Biophys Res Commun 2015;464(3):807–13.
30. Jasinski-Bergner S, Stoehr C, Bukur J, et al. Clinical relevance of miR-mediated HLA-G regulation and the associated immune cell infiltration in renal cell carcinoma. OncoImmunology 2015;4(6):e1008805.
31. Gao F, Zhao Z-L, Zhao W-T, et al. miR-9 modulates the expression of interferon-regulated genes and MHC class I molecules in human nasopharyngeal carcinoma cells. Biochem Biophys Res Commun 2013;431(3):610–6.

32. Hughes T, Adler A, Kelly JA, et al. Evidence for gene-gene epistatic interactions among susceptibility loci for systemic lupus erythematosus. Arthritis Rheum 2012;64(2):485–92.

33. Kirino Y, Bertsias G, Ishigatsubo Y, et al. Genome-wide association analysis identifies new susceptibility loci for Behçet's disease and epistasis between HLA-B*51 and ERAP1. Nat Genet 2013;45(2):202–7.

34. Cortes A, Pulit SL, Leo PJ, et al. Major histocompatibility complex associations of ankylosing spondylitis are complex and involve further epistasis with ERAP1. Nat Commun 2015;6:7146.

35. Lester S, McLure C, Williamson J, et al. Epistasis between the MHC and the RCA block in primary Sjogren syndrome. Ann Rheum Dis 2008;67(6):849–54.

36. Lester S, Stokes L, Skarratt KK, et al. Epistasis with HLA DR3 implicates the P2X7 receptor in the pathogenesis of primary Sjögren's syndrome. Arthritis Res Ther 2013;15(4):R71.

37. Castro-Santos P, Moro-García MA, Marcos-Fernández R, et al. ERAP1 and HLA-C interaction in inflammatory bowel disease in the Spanish population. Innate Immun 2017;23(5):476–81.

38. Moreno M, Silva EL, Ramirez LE, et al. Chagas' disease susceptibility/resistance: linkage disequilibrium analysis suggests epistasis between major histocompatibility complex and interleukin-10. Tissue Antigens 2004;64(1):18–24.

39. Zheng H-F, Zuo X-B, Lu W-S, et al. Variants in MHC, LCE and IL12B have epistatic effects on psoriasis risk in Chinese population. J Dermatol Sci 2011;61(2):124–8.

40. Harton J, Jin L, Hahn A, et al. Immunological functions of the membrane proximal region of MHC class II molecules. F1000Research 2016;5:368.

41. Barroso M, Tucker H, Drake L, et al. Antigen-B cell receptor complexes associate with intracellular major histocompatibility complex (MHC) class II molecules. J Biol Chem 2015;290(45):27101–12.

42. Lang P, Stolpa JC, Freiberg BA, et al. TCR-induced transmembrane signaling by peptide/MHC class II via associated Ig-alpha/beta dimers. Science 2001; 291(5508):1537–40.

43. Jin L, Waterman PM, Jonscher KR, et al. MPYS, a novel membrane tetraspanner, is associated with major histocompatibility complex class II and mediates transduction of apoptotic signals. Mol Cell Biol 2008;28(16):5014–26.

44. Babushok DV, Duke JL, Xie HM, et al. Somatic HLA mutations expose the role of class I–mediated autoimmunity in aplastic anemia and its clonal complications. Blood Adv 2017;1(22):1900–10.

45. McGranahan N, Rosenthal R, Hiley CT, et al. Allele-specific HLA loss and immune escape in lung cancer evolution. Cell 2017;171(6):1259–71.e11.

46. Hiraki A, Fuj N II, Murakami T, et al. High frequency of allele-specific down-regulation of HLA class I expression in lung cancer cell lines. Anticancer Res 2004; 24(3a):1525–8.

47. Nie Y. DNA hypermethylation is a mechanism for loss of expression of the HLA class I genes in human esophageal squamous cell carcinomas. Carcinogenesis 2001;22(10):1615–23.

48. Brea EJ, Oh CY, Manchado E, et al. Kinase regulation of human MHC class I molecule expression on cancer cells. Cancer Immunol Res 2016;4(11): 936–47.

49. Chang C-C, Pirozzi G, Wen S-H, et al. Multiple structural and epigenetic defects in the human leukocyte antigen class I antigen presentation pathway in a recurrent metastatic melanoma following immunotherapy. J Biol Chem 2015;290(44): 26562–75.

50. Mehta AM, Jordanova ES, Kenter GG, et al. Association of antigen processing machinery and HLA class I defects with clinicopathological outcome in cervical carcinoma. Cancer Immunol Immunother 2007;57(2):197–206.

51. Bandoh N, Ogino T, Katayama A, et al. HLA class I antigen and transporter associated with antigen processing downregulation in metastatic lesions of head and neck squamous cell carcinoma as a marker of poor prognosis. Oncol Rep 2010; 23(4):933–9.

52. Kamata Y, Kuhara A, Iwamoto T, et al. Identification of HLA class I-binding peptides derived from unique cancer-associated proteins by mass spectrometric analysis. Anticancer Res 2013;33(5):1853–9.

53. Nelde A, Schuster H, Kowalewski DJ, et al. Identification of naturally presented HLA ligands of enriched leukemic progenitor cells for peptide-based immunotherapy in Acute Myeloid Leukemia (AML). Blood 2016; 128(22):4046.

54. Berlin C, Kowalewski DJ, Schuster H, et al. Mapping the HLA ligandome landscape of acute myeloid leukemia: a targeted approach toward peptide-based immunotherapy. Leukemia 2015;29(3):647–59.

55. Neidert MC, Kowalewski DJ, Silginer M, et al. The natural HLA ligandome of glioblastoma stem-like cells: antigen discovery for T cell-based immunotherapy. Acta Neuropathol 2018;135(6):923–38.

56. Neumann A, Hörzer H, Hillen N, et al. Identification of HLA ligands and T-cell epitopes for immunotherapy of lung cancer. Cancer Immunol Immunother 2013; 62(9):1485–97.

57. Suda T, Tsunoda T, Daigo Y, et al. Identification of human leukocyte antigen-A24-restricted epitope peptides derived from gene products upregulated in lung and esophageal cancers as novel targets for immunotherapy. Cancer Sci 2007; 98(11):1803–8.

58. Kowalewski DJ, Schemionek M, Kanz L, et al. HLA ligandome analysis of Chronic Myeloid Leukemia (CML), revealed novel tumor associated antigens for peptide based immunotherapy. Stickel JS, ed. Blood 2013;122(21):3975.

59. Peper JK, Bösmüller H-C, Schuster H, et al. HLA ligandomics identifies histone deacetylase 1 as target for ovarian cancer immunotherapy. OncoImmunology 2016;5(5):e1065369.

60. Schuster H, Peper JK, Bösmüller H-C, et al. The immunopeptidomic landscape of ovarian carcinomas. Proc Natl Acad Sci 2017;114(46):E9942–51.

61. Marty R, Kaabinejadian S, Rossell D, et al. MHC-I genotype restricts the oncogenic mutational landscape. Cell 2017;171(6):1272–83.e15.

62. Chowell D, Morris LGT, Grigg CM, et al. Patient HLA class I genotype influences cancer response to checkpoint blockade immunotherapy. Science 2018; 359(6375):582–7.

63. Kellis M, Wold B, Snyder MP, et al. Defining functional DNA elements in the human genome. Proc Natl Acad Sci 2014;111(17):6131–8.

64. Casdagli M. Nonlinear prediction of chaotic time series. Physica D Nonlinear Phenomena 1989;35(3):335–56.

65. Grassberger P, Schreiber T, Schaffrath C. Nonlinear time sequence analysis. Int J Bifurcat Chaos 1991;1(3):521–47.

66. Provenzale A, Smith LA, Vio R, et al. Distinguishing between low-dimensional dynamics and randomness in measured time series. Physica D: Nonlinear Phenomena 1992;58(1–4):31–49.

67. Tsallis C. Dynamical scenario for nonextensive statistical mechanics. Physica A: Statistical Mechanics and its Applications 2004;340(1–3):1–10.

68. Karakatsanis LP, Pavlos GP, Iliopoulos AC, et al. Assessing information content and interactive relationships of subgenomic DNA sequences of the MHC using complexity theory approaches based on the non-extensive statistical mechanics. Physica A: Statistical Mechanics and its Applications 2018;505:77–93.

69. Floyd RA. Neuroinflammatory processes are important in neurodegenerative diseases: an hypothesis to explain the increased formation of reactive oxygen and nitrogen species as major factors involved in neurodegenerative disease development. Free Radic Biol Med 1999;26(9–10):1346–55.

70. Klegeris A, McGeer EG, McGeer PL. Therapeutic approaches to inflammation in neurodegenerative disease. Curr Opin Neurol 2007;20(3):351–7.

71. Yokoyama JS, Wang Y, Schork AJ, et al. Association between genetic traits for immune-mediated diseases and alzheimer disease. JAMA Neurol 2016; 73(6):691.

72. Jones L, Holmans PA, Hamshere ML, et al. Genetic evidence implicates the immune system and cholesterol metabolism in the aetiology of alzheimer's disease. El Khoury J, ed. PLoS One 2010;5(11):e13950.

Printed and bound by CPI Group (UK) Ltd, Croydon, CR0 4YY

03/10/2024

01040390-0011